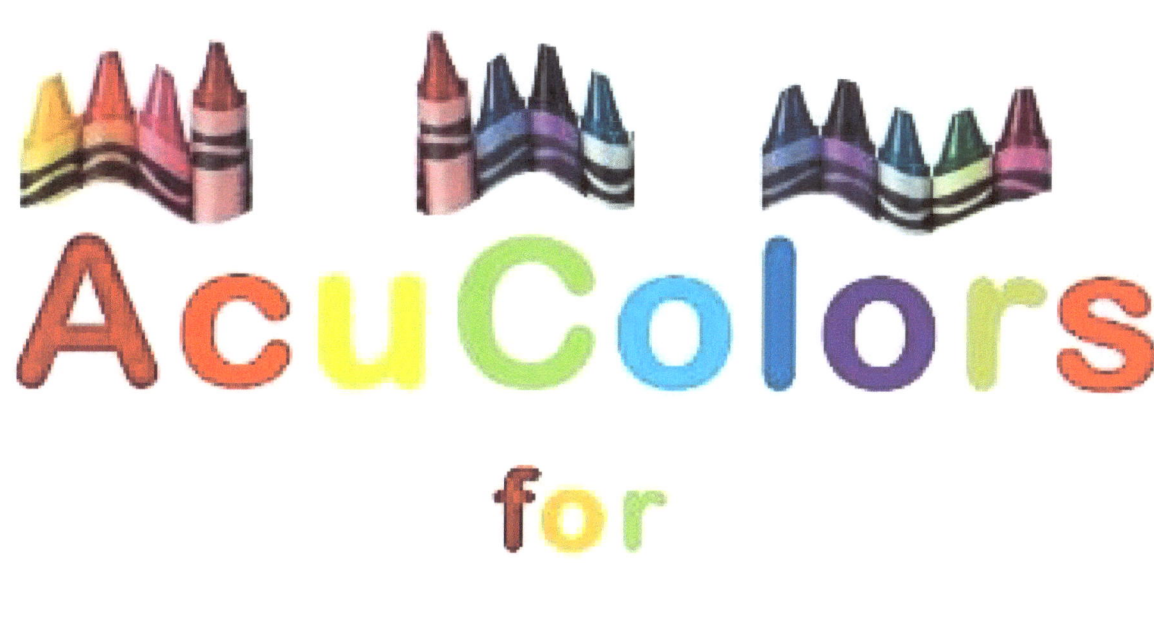

AcuColors for Animals

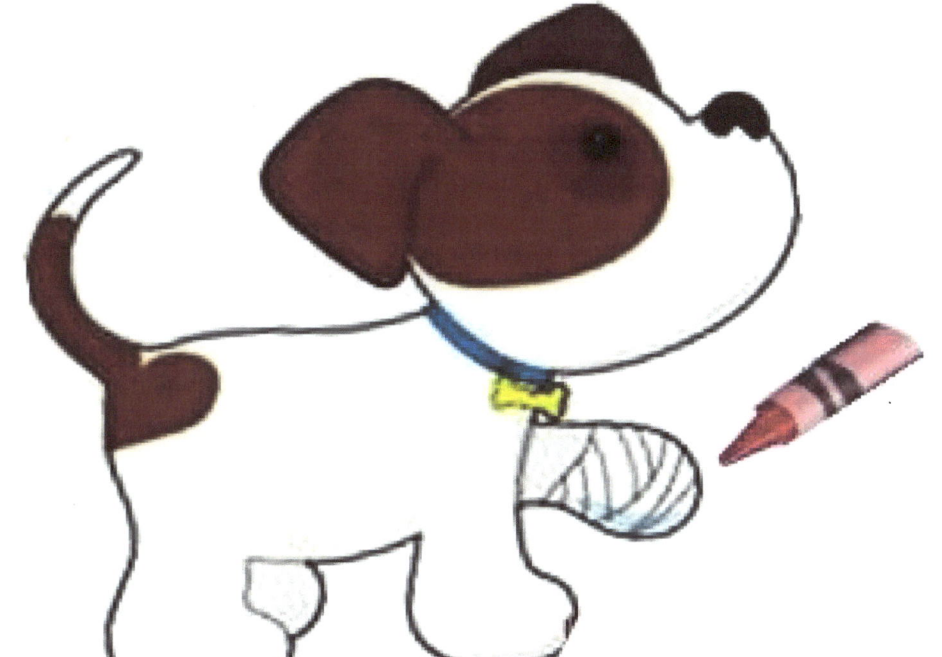

By Karen E Johnson, RN, MPH, CCP, Naturopath

AcuColors for Animals

By

Karen E Johnson, RN, MPH, CCP, Naturopath, Author

Walter W Johnson, Editor

www.AcuColors.com

Text copyright @ 2015 Karen E Johnson
ISBN: 9781520192291
2nd Edition

All rights reserved.

Without limiting the rights under copyright reserved above, no part of this publication may be reproduced, stored in or introduced into a retrieval system, or transmitted, in any form or by any means (electronic, mechanical, photocopying, recording or otherwise), without the prior written permission of both the copyright owner and the publisher of this book.

Published in the United States for Kindle eBook, 2015.

ACKNOWLEDGEMENTS

I must express my gratitude to my husband, Walter Johnson, for supporting me in my Esogetic Colorpuncture training, in the editing of this book, and in my Naturopathic school courses.

I greatly appreciate all of my clients for allowing me to share these skills while helping their pets.

DISCLAIMER

AcuColors does not provide medical advice, diagnosis or treatment.

Content from AcuColors is not intended to be used for medical diagnosis or treatment. The information provided in this book is intended for general consumer understanding and self-improvement only. The information provided is not intended to be a substitute for professional medical advice. As health and nutrition research continuously evolves, we do not guarantee the accuracy, completeness, or timeliness of any information presented in this book.

TABLE OF CONTENTS

ACKNOWLEDGEMENTS 3
DISCLAIMER 3
PREFACE 7
INTRODUCTION 9
    The Body 9
    The Soul 9
    The Spirit 10
    The Meridians 10
    5 Paired Meridian Pathways 11
PART I: ASSESSMENT GUIDE 13
PART II: THE 3 TREATMENT METHODS FOR HEALING THE BODY-SOUL-SPIRIT 16
SECTION 1: BODY SYSTEM REGULATORY TREATMENTS 18
    The Main Body Systems 18
    Body System Chart 19
    LYMPHATIC SYSTEM   LvGB 20
    NERVOUS SYSTEM   SpSt 21
    MUSCULOSKELETAL SYSTEM KiBl 22
    ENDOCRINE SYSTEM LuLI 24
    BLOOD IMMUNE SYSTEM   HtSI 26
SECTION II: A-Z SPECIAL HEALTH ISSUES 28
    Adrenal Fatigue (LuLI) 28
    Allergies, Skin (LuLI) 30
    Anger & Aggression (LvGB) 32
    Anxiety (KiBl) 33
    Arthritis (SpSt) 34
    Bladder / Urinary Issues (KiBl) 36
    Cancer (HtSI) 37
    Confusion (LvGB) 38
    Constipation (SpSt) 39
    Depression (LuLI) 40
    Diabetes (SpSt) 41
    Diarrhea (LuLI) 42
    Ear Disorders (KiBl) 43
    Epilepsy (HtSI) 44
    Eye disorders (LvGB) 45

Fear (KiBl)	46
Fever (HtSI)	47
Gastrointestinal Disorders (SpSt)	48
Heart-Lung Issues (HtSI)	49
Heat Stroke (HtSI)	50
Hip Dysplasia (SpSt)	51
Insomnia (HtSI)	52
Jaw Problems (SpSt)	53
Liver/Gall Bladder Problems (LvGB)	54
Pain	55
(HtSI)	55
Parasites (SpSt)	59
Neuter/Spay Recovery (LuLI)	60
Respiratory Problems (LuLI)	61
Reproduction Problems (LuLI)	62
Sadness or Grief (LuLI)	63
Sedation (KiBl)	64
Throat/Thyroid Conditions (LuLI)	65
Toothaches (LuLI)	66
Trauma, Emotional and Physical (HtSI)	67
SECTION III: BALANCING THE MERIDIANS	**68**
LIVER/GALL BLADDER MERIDIAN	71
STOMACH/SPLEEN MERIDIAN	72
KIDNEY/BLADDER MERIDIAN	73
LUNG/LARGE INTESTINE MERIDIAN	74
HEART/SMALL INTESTINE MERIDIAN	75
CONCLUSION	**76**
APPENDIX 1: FINDING THE RIGHT COLOR TOOLS	**77**
APPENDIX 3: DENTAL CONNECTION	**82**
APPENDIX 2: EFFECTS OF COLOR	**83**
APPENDIX 6: PET CPR & FIRST AID	**87**
APPENDIX 4: SPINAL CONNECTION	**90**
APPENDIX 5: GROOMING GUIDE	**91**
GLOSSARY	**93**
REFERENCES	**95**

PREFACE

Traditional Chinese Medicine (TCM) teaches us not to chase after symptoms, but to regulate the body systems, remove emotional blockages, and rebalance the "meridian" energy pathways of the body.

The use of color on the acupuncture points (acupoints) of the body is every bit as, and perhaps even more, effective as acupuncture; because the color actually penetrates deeper into the body's cells. Acucolors does not introduce sources of infection from needles, and has no side effects. Occasionally there may be symptoms from a "healing cycle" that subside within 24 hours. These symptoms are actually a good sign that your body is responding to the treatment by releasing an emotion and healing the cells. Most of the time you will feel nothing, except the overall improvement.

Here are some tips for working with Acucolors that show just how straightforward the following the treatment protocols can be:

- **Intent**: In using any of TCM's techniques it's all about *intent*. If you have the intent to heal your pet, he will heal.

- **Placement**: The placement of color on the acupoints doesn't have to be exact, especially using a bigger diameter of your color penlight. To check location of an acupoint, probe for a soft tissue depression or hole between the hard boney structures that most likely will be *tender or sore*. The length of time for color placement doesn't have to be super accurate; but a minimum of 15-20 seconds per point is recommended.

- **Longer Treatment Protocols**: Some of the treatment protocols have more acupoints than others. If your time is limited try just treating the acupoints that address the areas of most concern. For example, in the case of Asthma, you could just treat points #1 & 3 in the chart below. Additional points are given, because they are part of the protocol in treating the affected meridians. It is best to do the complete treatment, but it's better to do something rather than nothing.

Pts	Acupoint & Location	Acupoint Indications	Color
1.	**CV22** in hole above sternum	Cough, Asthma, Sore throat, Goiter, Chest pain	Red
2.	**Lu5** L&R inside front leg middle elbow crease	Bronchitis, Pneumonia, Cough, Dyspnea	L-Blue R-Orange
3.	**Lu7** L&R inside front leg just above radial wrist joint	Asthma, cough, neck, toothache	L-Blue R-Orange

- **Negative emotions**: Negative emotions aren't necessarily released in a dramatic way with the physical symptom dissipating into thin air. It may take time and persistence in repeating the specific treatments. The preferred pattern for any color treatment is: *once a day for a week, once a week for a month, once a month for a year.* The physical symptoms won't return with perseverance.

- **Color Frequencies**: Color is color. Don't be overly concerned about exact color frequencies in selecting your color tools. Use the green shade you feel will heal infections and complement red. If it's all you have, using a Blue-Violet and Red laser pen on acupoints is better than not using any color. Suggestions for inexpensive color tools are made in [Appendix 2](#).

One tool that works well with Acucolors is Dr. Bradley Nelson's *Emotion Code*. I use this often for my dog, Ricki. When he was a puppy he had Parvo and almost didn't survive. This traumatic event alone has caused much worry and fear in Ricki. He exhibits behaviors such as hiding under the bed so he won't get caught for a bath. These acute little worries can turn into chronic anxieties and even become embedded as fears, if not released. By regularly testing for emotions using the Emotion Code techniques Ricki is saved from unnecessary physical hardships.

Learning Emotion Code is based on muscle testing. Dr. Nelson charted 60 basic emotions and categorized them into meridian pairs. Simply release the negative emotions swiping a magnet down the spine at least 3-5x; and then by balancing the meridian pairs. ([Pt II Section 3](#))

INTRODUCTION

AcuColors' use of colored light on the acupuncture points (acupoints) not only draws the Physical Body's own healing powers to cellular locations that need repair, but it also releases negative emotions from the Soul and clears the energy pathways or meridians of the Spirit.

Our 4-legged pets cannot tell us subjectively what's bothering them, this book will address the objective signs that you as a pet owner can see; and then suggest color treatments that will help you identify negative emotions and physical ailments in your cat, dog, pig, horse, etc. Using these treatments you may be able to heal them in a pain-free loving manner in the home environment without the stress to you or your pet of visiting the Vet. The added benefit of this approach is the bonding that can take place with your pet, like the bonding that can occur when you groom your pet yourself instead of dropping them off at the Groomer.

Let me relate an experience with my little Shitzu/Poodle to illustrate why it is important to identify and treat negative emotions in animals early on. Ricki is a small nervous dog, full of fear—mainly fear of my daughter's 2 year old Labrador "monster", Jinx who lives in the backyard. Jinx doesn't understand why he has to stay outside while his buddy gets to come inside with us, so in his jealousy he bats Ricki around and treats him like one of his play toys. In Ricki's eyes, every time he goes out to use the backyard facilities, he gets tortured. Imagine the anxiety and even fear that could build up in a situation like this, possibly even leading to physical issues if not dealt with in a timely manner. Negative emotions of fear, anger, worry and sadness can lead to physical problems if not addressed.

This book will discuss simple methods to release these negative emotions, treat physical issues, and balance the "meridians" of the body. This book will help improve communication between the Body-Soul-Spirit of our special pets such as Ricki, so that they remain happy and healthy.

That brings us to the concepts of Body, Soul, and Spirit. ...

The Body

The Body is the physical *vector,* or vessel, which contains the Soul and the Spirit. It needs nutrition and exercise to remain healthy and functional. It is subject to physical harm from accident or illness.

The Soul

The Soul is the psychological *reflector* of emotion. It can be portrayed as an aura around the outside of the body. Emotions can be reflected outward, and some people can see them, even in spectral colors, as a glow around the body.

Do you have a pet that you totally connect with? Maybe you feel that you can read your pet's mind, or that your pet can read yours? The emotional auras between people and their pets can blend together making it easier to feel what the other is feeling. Emotional auras can also repel each other, much like a pair of magnets can attract each other in one orientation, or repel each other in the opposite. Have you ever met a dog that you instantly fell in love with, as opposed to one that you knew was dangerous to you?

The Soul also supports instinctive drives for love and satisfaction of physical needs which are for the most part, housed in the gut. Animals are basically driven by their instinct or "gut feelings".

The Spirit

Every living being has a spirit. The Spirit is the rational, intellectual *director*, or in other words, the mind. The spirit can take control of the body allowing one to press forward in spite of fear or of physically injury. As an example, think of all the times you have heard of pets warning their owners of danger, or even of putting themselves at risk by rescuing their owners from situations like burning buildings. In this case, the mind spirit overrides the soul, or the gut instinctive feeling that the burning building is potentially harmful.

The Spirit MUST communicate properly with the Soul or conflict can arise in the form of physiological harm. As mentioned above, when two auras overlap or connect, the Soul helps the Spirit interpret the information it receives. For example, the Soul can feel whether the other person is really mad or just kidding, which helps the Spirit know how to react.

The Meridians

Valuable information is distributed throughout the whole body-soul-spirit being by way of an energy pathway system. The spirit is located at the center of this meridian pathway system. Meridians are energy pathways that carry information from the Spirit to the Soul and to the Body. Communication through this energy network is as essential to survival as the flow of blood through the circulatory network. The body would be lifeless without the information it receives from this meridian pathway system

AcuColors can repair damage to the meridian's energy network by regulating body systems, releasing physical or emotional blockages, and by rebalancing the meridian pathways.

> *When you heal a blocked meridian point you can repair and balance its whole energy pathway. Perfect health then, could be defined as having all your meridians unblocked.*

Now, Let's put this altogether
This *illustration* gives a conceptual idea of the paired meridian pathways for a dog.

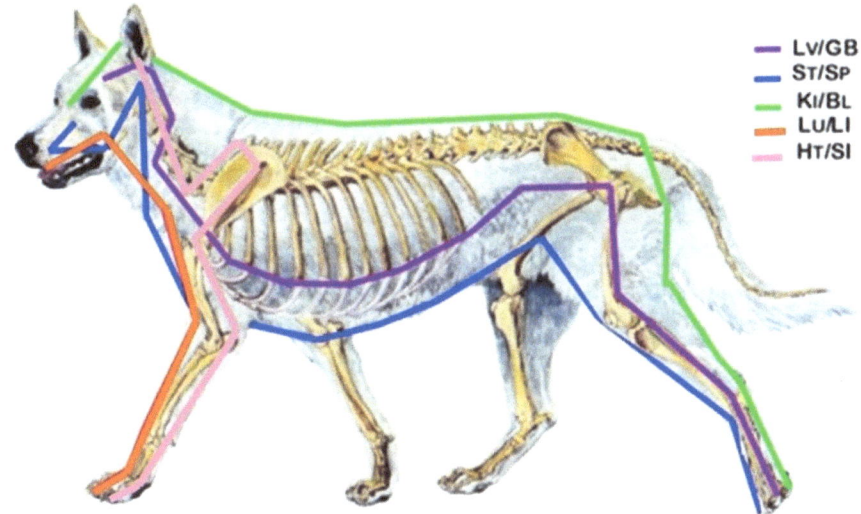

There are 10 major organs of the body with related meridian pathways. These become 5 paired meridians when combined with their yin/yang opposites. For example: The Liver is paired with the Gallbladder and their predominant emotion together is anger. Together they have various physical disease tendencies.

The chart below lists these 5 paired meridians with their associated emotion and diseases. If you have identified a negative emotion in your pet, such as anger, you may have also observed some physical issues listed in the chart, such as allergies. Complete healing of your pet would involve using color to:

1. regulate the flow of the lymphatic system (Pt II, Sec 1)
2. release the anger while addressing the specific health issue of allergies (Pt II, Sec 2), and
3. rebalance the Liver/Gall Bladder meridians (Pt II, Sec 3).

The longer you wait to release the anger, the more difficult it becomes to heal your pet from the associated physical disease such as allergies. You might notice that some of the physical disease tendencies are listed under more than one meridian. This is because those meridian pathways run closely together in especially the face and neck where allergies are triggered. In this case, you should balance both Lv/GB and Lu/LI meridians. (See Part II, Sec 3)

5 Paired Meridian Pathways

SPIRITUAL MERIDIAN NETWORK	MAIN SOUL EMOTION	PHYSICAL DISEASE TENDENCIES OF THE BODY
Liver/Gall Bladder Lv/GB	Anger	Allergies, Anxiety, Convulsions, Dizziness, Eye & Ear issues, Fever, Hip pain or Arthritis, Hypertension, Mood disorders, Muscle Atrophy, Nausea, Numbness, Rib pain, Shoulder pain, Stroke, Weakness
Stomach/Spleen	Worry	Anemia, Anorexia, Diabetes, Food Poisoning, Glaucoma, Joint & Bone

St/Sp		pain, Knee pain, Nausea, Toothache, Urinary Tract infections
Kidney/Bladder Ki/Bl	Fear	Anorexia, Arthritis, Bladder infections, Edema, Epilepsy, Fatigue, Back paw pain, Hearing; Joint pain, Knee, Leg, Low Back Pain, Muscle spasms, Osteoporosis, Premature Graying, Rapid Pulse, Hereditary weaknesses, Respiratory ailments, Systemic diseases, Urinary disorders
Lung/Large Intestine Lu/LI	Sadness	==Allergies==, Asthma, Bronchitis, Cold/Flu, Congestion, Depression, Diarrhea, Dry Skin, Eczema, Elbow pain, Fatigue, Itching, Sneezing, Sore throat, Stress, Toothache.
Heart/Small Intestine Ht/SI	Love	Anemia, Blood Pressure/Heart rate & rhythm, Cough; Shoulder & Neck pain. Sore Throat, Fatigue, Insomnia, Mouth sores, Neuralgia, Nightmares. Fever, Sweating, Swollen Glands.

So how do we know if our pet has any of these physical disease tendencies since they can't communicate very easily with us? Use the following assessment guide in Part I to help find clues and to better understand your pet's specific needs.

PART I: ASSESSMENT GUIDE

Start out with a full head-to-toe assessment of your pet using this 10-point guide in the chart below. The assessment guide lists the overall affected meridians that go along with the signs observed. So, in order to treat a specific problem such as itchy ears which could indicate an ear infection and is listed as an issue in the KiBl meridian, do:
1. the Regulatory treatment for the KiBl (Kidney Bladder meridian) which is the Musculoskeletal regulation treatment. (Pt II, Sec 1)
2. the Ear Disorder specific treatment to remove emotional blockages (Pt II, Sec 2)
3. the rebalancing of the Kidney Bladder meridians. (Pt II, Sec 3)

Weekly assessments while grooming your pet can help avoid a pattern of imbalance that leads to illness. See Grooming Guide in Appendix 5.

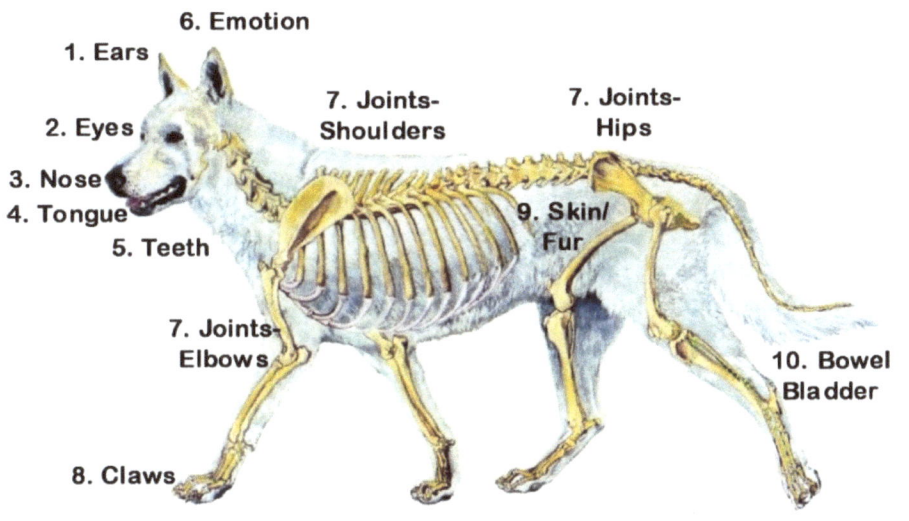

	Body Part/System	Sign Observed	Special Note
1.	**EARS** KiBl	**Infection** Scratching at ear, Odor, Shaking of Head, Ear Pain, Debris in Ear (Mites) **Hearing Loss**--No response to Loud Noise	
2.	**EYES** LvGB	**Infection**--Yellow or Green Discharge Dull Red sticky eyelids Yellow Eyes--Jaundice **Vision Loss**--Squinting No Response to Visual Cues Inactivity due to Diminished Sight Compensates loss using other senses more	**See Vet**: If extremely Red under lids or on White of eye. Yellow or Green discharge. No response to visual cues.
3.	**NOSE** & Respiratory system LuLI	Dry Sneezing Sinus congestion Hot or Cold	**See Vet**: If Nose Hot & Dry. Runny discharge. Dry cough that doesn't go away.
4.	**TEETH/MOUTH** & Digestive system	Dirty, Stained, Worn or Broken, Difficulty Chewing, Gums Inflamed. See Appendix 3	**See Vet**: If Won't eat nor drink. Throws

	SpSt	for info on individual teeth and the meridian connection.	up repeatedly. Foaming at mouth
5.	**TONGUE**: Look at color & coating. Color reflects circulation in the body. Normal should be all pink no cracks, clear coating **HtSI** 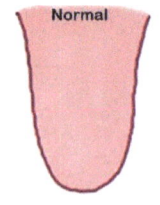	**Lv/GB: Anger** 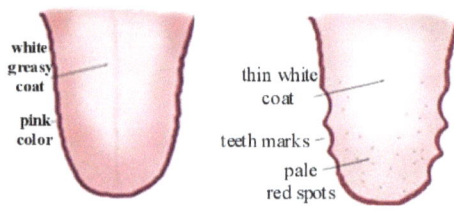 **Sp/St: Worry** 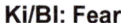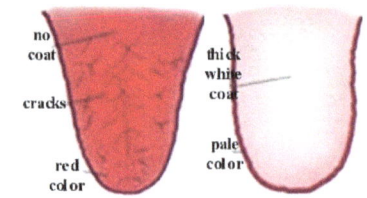 **Ki/Bl: Fear** **Lu/LI: Sadness** 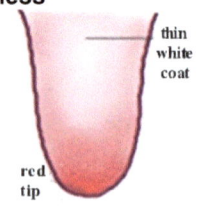	The color of the tongue can show meridian blockages or hidden emotions that need releasing.

	EMOTION		
6.	**Anger** (Lv/GB = 11p-3a*)	Snarls or Growls	
	Worry (Sp/St = 7a-11a*)	Resists new situations or change	
	Fear (Ki/Bl = 3p-7p*)	Hides out	
	Betrayal (Ht/SI = 11a-3p*)	Won't get up	
7.	**JOINTS**—Hip, Shoulder, Elbows	Limited mobility Severe pain Stiff Joints	**See Vet**: If Favors Hip, Shoulder,

	KiBl	Hot Swollen Joints	Elbow & will not bear weight Noticeable Dislocation of Bone or Joint
8.	**CLAWS** **LuLl**	Broken or Cracked	**See Vet**: If Bleeding & Painful while walking
9.	**SKIN** **LuLl**	Fur uneven or unclean Red Inflamed Itchy Hot Spots Loss of Fur or Dander Brittle Dry Dull Coat Fleas, Ticks, Blisters, Raised Rash Scabs	**See Vet**: If Sarcoptic or Didactic Mange Dehydration—skin doesn't retract when pinched.
10	**BOWEL** LuLl **BLADDER** KiBl	Diarrhea or Soft Stool Fecal Impaction Anal glands full—infected or impacted Loss of Bladder Control Leaking or Dribbling	**See Vet**: If Diarrhea > 24 hrs Very stinky dark scant urine

*Note the time of day for peak meridian activity.

The treatments in *AcuColors for Animals* are presented in an easy-to-follow "recipe" format to help anyone understand how to heal their pet on the whole body-soul-spirit levels.

The AcuColors regulatory treatments in Part II, Section 1 address lymphatic detoxification, nervous system and musculoskeletal disorders, endocrine imbalances, and immune system issues. Section 2 addresses specific physical health issues. Section III covers realigning the meridian pathways to maintain a healthy state.

It is important to begin by treating the basic body regulation first, discussed in Part I, Section 1. Many times simply treating the glandular and lymphatic dysfunction is sufficient to maintain the good health of your pet. If special health issues exist, refer to Section 2. Finally, when your pet is more stable emotionally and physically, move on to Section 3: *Balancing the Meridians* to ensure that your pet stays healthy.

PART II: THE 3 TREATMENT METHODS FOR HEALING THE BODY-SOUL-SPIRIT

1. **Section 1: <u>Body Level</u>: The Regulatory Treatments** resynchronize the physical body systems, moderate mood swings, and reduce the likelihood of unwanted emotions.

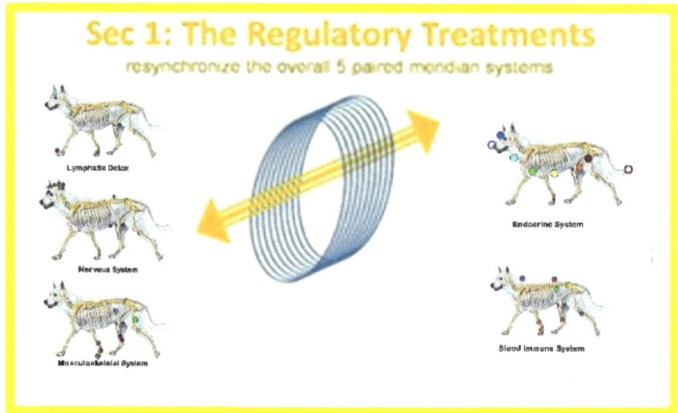

2. **Section 2: <u>Soul Level</u>: Treatments for Specific Health Issues** -- release buried negative emotions in targeted organs.

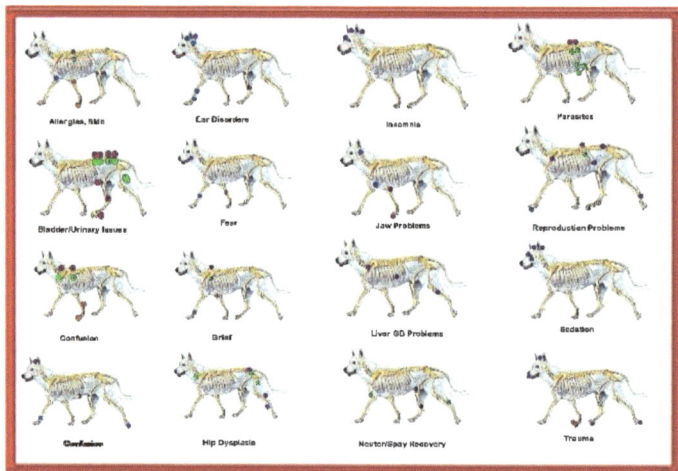

3. **Section 3: <u>Spirit Level</u>: Meridian Balancing** --Tracing the energy pathways rebalances the meridians curing disease.

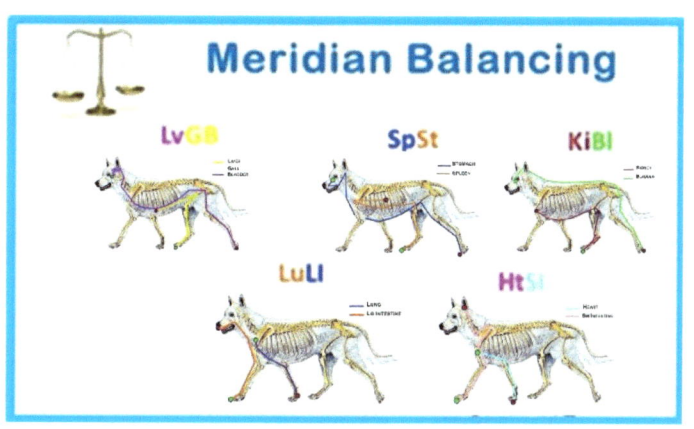

SECTION 1: BODY SYSTEM REGULATORY TREATMENTS

Disease patterns occur from dysregulation of body processes. The body is always trying to heal itself and usually succeeds until dysregulation breaks down cell communication. The disease process is like walking down a hallway that becomes narrower with each step. Fortunately, most of the time, the disease process is slow and according to Constantine Hering's law, begins from bottom to top; outside to inside; from the lesser organs, like the skin, to the greater organs, like the heart. Healing begins in the reverse order so the greatest organ—the heart—is often spared any damage since it is the last to be affected by disease and the first to be repaired from healing.

The following basic treatments work on the physical body level to restore regulation and balance to each of these main body systems, and they should be utilized prior to any of the treatments in the next two sections of this book.

The Main Body Systems

The *Lymphatic system*, represented by the Dewclaws or (1st) claws, is essential in removing toxic waste from the body. About 10% of the blood plasma becomes lymph fluid for removal of waste. The tonsils, adenoids, spleen and thymus are important parts of the lymphatic system. The Liver and Kidneys eliminate most of the toxic waste.

The *Nerve-Musculoskeletal systems*, represented by the 2nd and 3rd claws, provide the body's ability to move. For many reasons the nerves, muscles, bones and connective tissues degenerate making movement difficult. Degeneration occurs when the body sees joints, muscles, connective tissue, glands and organs as foreign. Antibodies are then produced against it causing pain and inflammation. When you have one autoimmune issue it's not uncommon to have multiple. Autoimmunity begins much of the time as a result of an allergy. Over the years food has been altered for reasons beyond our control. Wheat seed has already been genetically modified leading to gluten intolerances in the gut. If the gut doesn't recognize altered food, it naturally treats it as a foreign substance building antibodies against it. There is no other solution but to get back to the basics of eating unaltered grains.

The *Endocrine system*, represented by the 4th claws, controls the glandular function. Each gland is directly related to a chakra energy center which must be aligned for the glands to function properly. The Thyroid is one of most important glands; without it, the body would not survive. Airborne or foodborne allergens introduced to the body through the Lung or Intestinal systems weaken the endocrine glands. These glands influence a person on the psychological and physical levels; so can you imagine what happens when there is not only Lung or Colon disease, but poor glandular function? The Endocrine treatment given in this section will realign the chakras and help the associated glands and organ systems to function better.

The *Blood Circulatory & Immune defense system*, represented by the 5th claws, is run by the Autonomic Nervous System without conscious effort. There is only one heart and one small intestine so all other organs and meridians pathways must protect it for survival. Proverbs 4:23 says "Guard your heart above everything else because from it flow the issues of life." The thinking, feeling, beating power of the heart is essential to the health of the whole man. The heart links the body-soul-spirit and is the central most important organ of the body.

Body System Chart

BODY SYSTEM	Lymphatic Lv GB	Nervous Sp St	Musc Skel Ki Bl	Endocrine Lu LI	Immune Ht SI
CLAW	R & L 1st Dewclaw	R & L 2nd	R & L 3rd	R & L 4th	R & L 5th
REGULATING FUNCTION	Immune support & eliminate toxins thru lymphatic system.	Transfer info between nerves & muscles for movement	Transfer info between nerves & muscles for movement	Gland & Hormone Regulation	Circulation of oxygenated blood to the vital cells & organs
PROBLEM	Congestion	Degeneration	Degeneration	Dysregulation	Stagnation

THE ROLE OF THE LYMPHATIC & ENDOCRINE SYSTEMS together is to protect the Heart & Small Intestine at all costs & to prevent degeneration of the nervous and musculoskeletal systems. Treat the Lymphatic and Endocrine claws <u>first</u>. Finally, approach the other body systems until they become balanced as well.

LYMPHATIC SYSTEM   LvGB

Where there is pain, swelling and inflammation, there is toxicity from poor lymphatic drainage. Detoxifying the body will relieve pain, inflammation, allergies, sinusitis and all congestion.

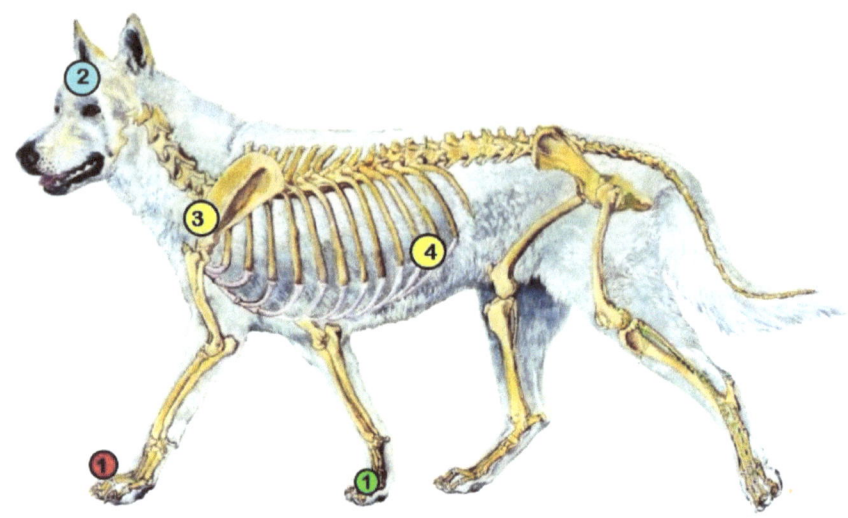

DETOXIFICATION

1.	Location	Indications	Color
2.	LI4 L&R inside forepaw in web between dewclaw & toe 1	Immune mediated skin issues. Sore throat, Cough, Neck, Shoulder pain, Lameness, Fever. Not for PG	L-Green R-Red
3.	GV21 mid Forehead at level of bottom of ears	Epilepsy, ADHD, Sinus Congestion	Turquoise
4.	Lu1 L&R base of neck before 1st rib	Cough, Asthma, Tension	Yellow
5.	Lv13 L&R at lowest point 12th rib on sides	Fatigue, Abdominal pain & Distention, Swelling of legs	Yellow

General Indications: For Sinus, Liver & Lymphatic Congestion, Pain & Swelling of Legs, Shoulders from injuries or illness.

Directions: Start with Point 1 on both front feet in Red/Green complementary color balance. Shine light 15-20 seconds per point. Proceed with Point 2 on forehead. Points 3 & 4 are on both Left & Right sides.

♪ **Reflexology**: To improve Lymphatic drainage and improve CNS function. Use Foot Reflexology Yellow on underside of back paw. Violet on top part of back paw. Stroke lines back & forth 30 seconds each on both back paws.

NERVOUS SYSTEM   SpSt

The Vagus is the longest cranial nerve running all the way from the head down to the colon, controlling everything from brain function, heart and lungs, to digestion and elimination.

The following treatment balances the Nervous system.

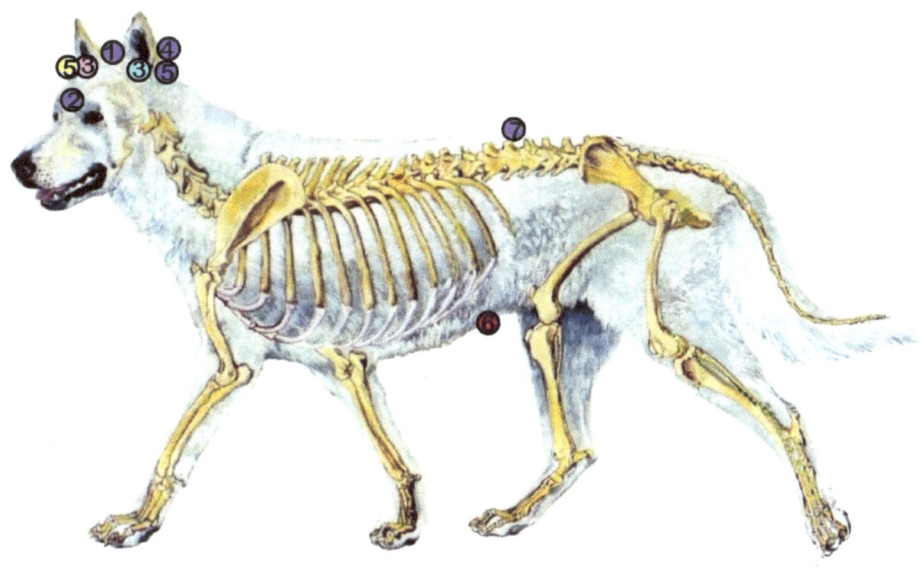

	Point & Location	Acupoint Indication	Color
1	**GV20** top head; straight ↑ from top of ears	Aphasia, insomnia, memory, HA, Tinnitus, Vertigo	Violet
2	**GV24.5 Yin Trang** or **Pineal** between eyebrows	Insomnia	Violet
3	**SI19** Hairline front of ear	Insomnia, intolerance to heat & cold; appetite, fatigue, memory, BP	L Turquoise R Pink *
4	**GV19** mid ridge on back crown of head	Seizure, HA, Dizziness, Mental disorders	Violet
5	**GB20 Medulla pts** at L&R corners of back hairline	Epilepsy, HA, Vertigo, Tinnitus, Stroke, Face palsy, LBP, NP, Eye Redness & Pain	L Violet R Yellow
6	**CV6** 2FW↓Navel	Stroke, GERD, abd pain, dysentery, constipation, enuresis, dysuria, impotence, PMS, prolapse uterus & rectum	Red
7	**GV3** on L5/S1 Medulla pt	LBP, Muscle atrophy & Leg Pain, PMS, Impotence	Violet

*If Pink is unavailable, use orange.

General Indications: Nervous System degenerative disorders such as—Balance, Palsy or anything that affects memory and ability to perform daily activities.

Directions: Apply appropriate colors for 20 seconds each.

MUSCULOSKELETAL SYSTEM KiBl

The skeleton provides solid structure for locomotion, stores minerals and lipids; produces red blood cells and protects the organs. The muscles provide movement, posture, joint stability and heat production. Considering how much force and weight we place on our body's structure, it's amazing it doesn't degenerate faster.

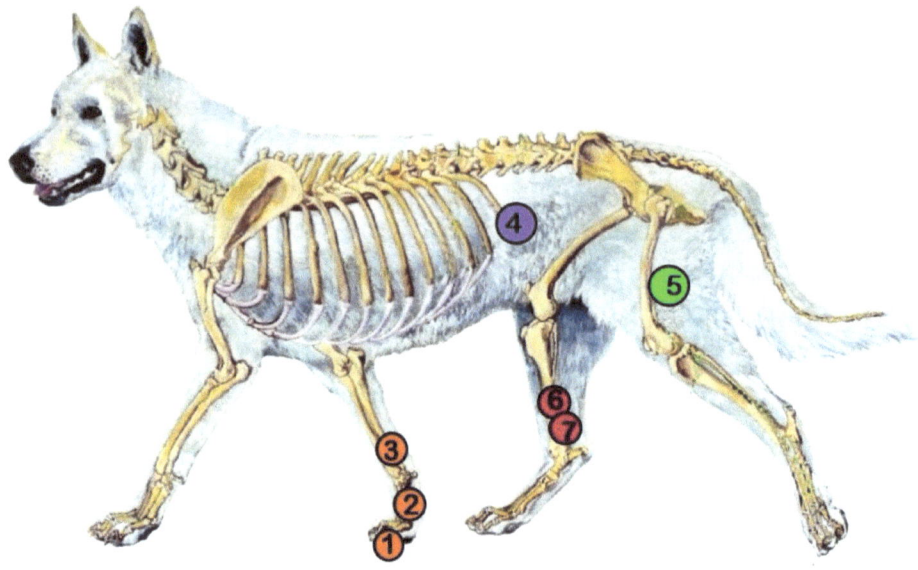

Signs: n/v, passing only small amounts of urine; swelling ankles; fatigue; loss of appetite; itchy; limps, refuses to stand up; favors leg; complains of pain when petting head or back.

	Location	Indications	Color
1.	**LI4** L&R inside forepaw in web between dewclaw & toe 1	Immune mediated skin issues. Sore throat, Cough, Neck, Shoulder pain, Lameness, Fever. Not for PG	L-Blue R-Orange
2.	**Lu7** L&R inside front leg just above radial wrist joint	Asthma, cough, neck, toothache	L-Blue R-Orange
3.	**TH3** L&R inside front paw 1FW↑joint	Eye & ear issues, fever, shoulder pain	L-Turquoise R-Orange
4.	**GB25** L&R end of 13th rib on side of body	Abdominal or LBP, water metabolism disorders, Expels Kidney stones	L-Violet R-Yellow
5.	**Bl40** L&R on outside & backside of hindleg where it meets body.	LBP, Hips, Stifles, incontinence, AI disorders, spondylosis, paralysis	L-Green R-Red
6.	**K7** L&R 2FW↑ K3 above hock on inside hindleg	Kidney &LBP, edema, diarrhea, paralysis	L-Green R-Red
7.	**K3** L&R 1FW↑ inside hindleg hock	Arthritis, local swelling of hock, LBP, Kidney, ear issues	L-Green R-Red

General Indications: For edema, fear, kidney stones, hearing issues, LBP; most any body system can be affected by kidney problems.

Directions: Shine colored light 15-20 seconds per point.

ENDOCRINE SYSTEM LuLl

EACH CHAKRA is linked to a gland. *When you balance the chakra you help regulate the gland.* Also, significant emotional trauma is imprinted in the Chakras; so *when you balance the Chakras,* **you release negative emotions.**

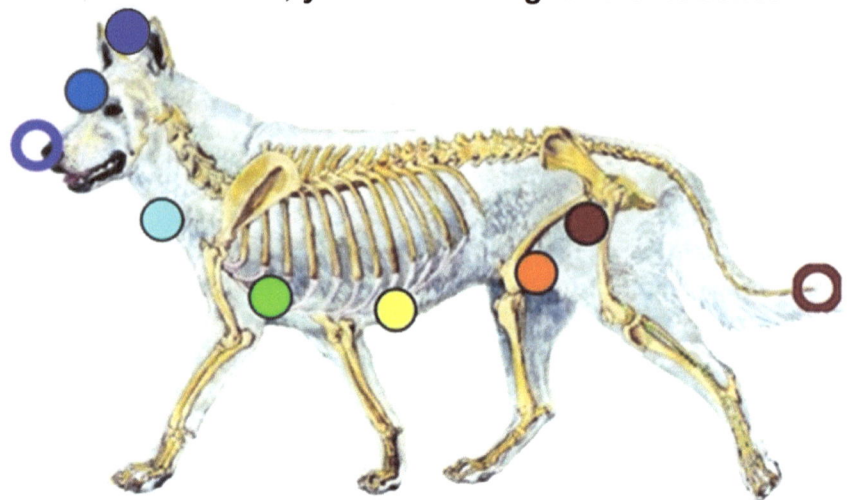

CHAKRA BALANCING

Chakra	Point & Location	Gland	Function	Color
Earth	Tail Tip	Adrenals	Survival	Red
Root	CV1 mid anus & vulva or scrotum	Adrenals	Survival	Red
Sacral	CV4 4FW↓ navel	Gonads	Create	Orange
Solar Plexus	CV12 midway from xyphoid to navel	Pancreas	Satisfy	Yellow
Heart	CV18 Mid sternum	Thymus	Share	Green
Throat	On throat	Thyroid	Communicate	Turquoise
Brow	Yin Trang between eyebrows	Pineal	Wholeness	Indigo
Crown	GV20 top head; ↑ from top of ears	Pituitary	Intuition	Violet
Crown	Nose Tip	**Pituitary**	**Intuition**	**Ultraviolet**

General Indications: For Endocrine disorders—Thyroid, Adrenal glands, Autoimmune and Metabolic Disorders

Directions: I have included two secondary chakras—the tip of the tail & the nose since some practitioners feel these are major chakras, when in reality they are extensions of the major root and crown chakras. Starting at the Tail (Infrared) & Root Chakra (Red), place appropriate color on each Chakra for 20 sec. During each light placement, use a swirling or circular motion clockwise around that part of the body where the light is placed. Check for movement of the Chakras by holding a clear or appropriately colored crystal on a string above the chakra. Watch for movement of the crystal. The faster it spins the more balanced the chakra. The Chakras can spin in either direction, but Clockwise is preferred since the energy tends to move outward and join other energy; while Counter Clockwise moves energy inward and tends to drain other energy. If one of the chakras will not move, swirl the colored light longer until it does. If there is still no movement, then suspect blockage(s). Look at the Gland and its Function in the chart above. If you know your pet already has issues with that gland, then this is further confirmation that you need to work with it to unblock the corresponding chakra.

BLOOD IMMUNE SYSTEM   HtSI

When serious skin conditions develop, such as Sarcoptic Mange, it is very difficult to stop the progression of the disease, once it has become systemic. Early Detection of Systemic Diseases through weekly and monthly assessments is essential to the longevity of life of your pet. This treatment will help your pet's immune system fight against serious degenerative diseases. A few years ago, I had the unfortunate experience of watching my rescue pet, Wolfie, suffer with Sarcoptic Mange and I wish I had had this information to save him, but unfortunately, the age and background of the pet also plays into his longevity of life as well.

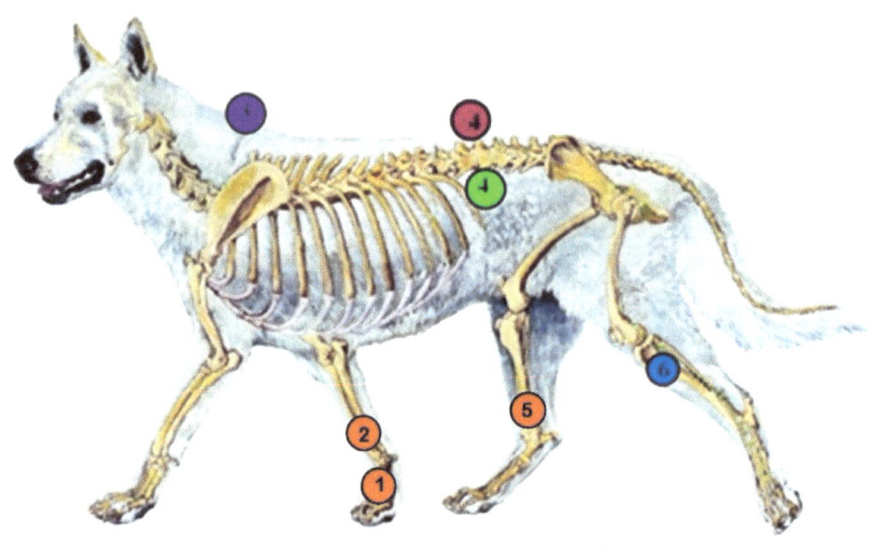

	Location	Indications	Color
1.	**LI4** L&R inside forepaw in web between dewclaw & toe 1	Immune mediated skin issues. Sore throat, Cough, Neck, Shoulder pain, Lameness, Fever. Not for PG	L-Blue R-Orange
2.	**Lu7** L&R just above radial wrist joint	Asthma, cough, neck, toothache	L-Blue R-Orange
3.	**GV14** between C7 &T1 on spine	Fever, cough, cervical pain, spondylosis, immune system.	Violet
4.	**Bl23** 3FW each side of L2	Weakness, seizures, ears, eyes, LBP, kidney, focus, brain	L-Green R-Red
5.	**Sp6** L&R inside hindleg 3FW↑ hock	Hypothyroidism, edema, fatigue, incontinence, immune, not for PG	L-Blue R-Orange
6.	**St36** L&R 1FW↓knee joint hind legs	Stomach, ulcers, constipation, diarrhea, weakness. Not for PG	L-Blue R-Orange

General Indications: For Systemic diseases, Autoimmune disorders, Muscle-Nerve degeneration, Skin conditions-Sarcoptic or Didactic Mange, Cancer. These Acupoints work together to boost the immune system, and additionally help with the indications noted in the above table.

Directions: Shine colored light 15-20 seconds per point.

- Frankincense essential oil helps fight cancer and other systemic diseases.

SECTION II: A-Z SPECIAL HEALTH ISSUES

The beauty of AcuColors is that lighted color enters the cells at the body level and directly heals the body. Whatever is unneeded by the body is not utilized. So, in essence, any color, any placement restores health to the body. There are no side effects whatsoever. The following color treatments are directed to specific health issues, listed in alphabetical order.

Adrenal Fatigue (LuLI)

Adrenal Fatigue is not often recognized by Endocrinologists and it can occur in humans or animals. This state is in between overstimulation or constant Fight or Flight (called "Cushing's disease), and when the adrenal glands actually wear down to little or no stimulation (Addison's disease). If the adrenal glands are allowed to overproduce cortisol (the Fight or Flight hormone) symptoms occur such as—insomnia, heart palpitations, anxiety, memory loss. The cortisol level may not be high enough to be classified as Cushing's disease, so a saliva test measuring the ASI (adrenal stress index) was created. This test also measures other indicators such as the DHEA, Fasting Insulin, Progesterone, IgA (immunocytes), and Gliadin (Gluten intolerance) and is beneficial in estimating where you are on that middle road of adrenal fatigue. The opposite end of the spectrum is Addison's disease, which is extreme end stage adrenal failure. Now, why the docs want to wait to recognize that you have little or no adrenal function until you are on your death bed, I'll never know! Symptoms of low adrenal function are salt craving, low blood pressure, extreme fatigue, hair loss, dizziness, depression, no libido, cold or heat intolerance. A good reference on Adrenal Fatigue is by Dr. James Wilson. http://www.amazon.com/Adrenal-Fatigue-Century-Stress-Syndrome/dp/1890572152/ref=sr_1_1?ie=UTF8&qid=1439994696&sr=8-1&keywords=dr+wilson+adrenal+fatigue

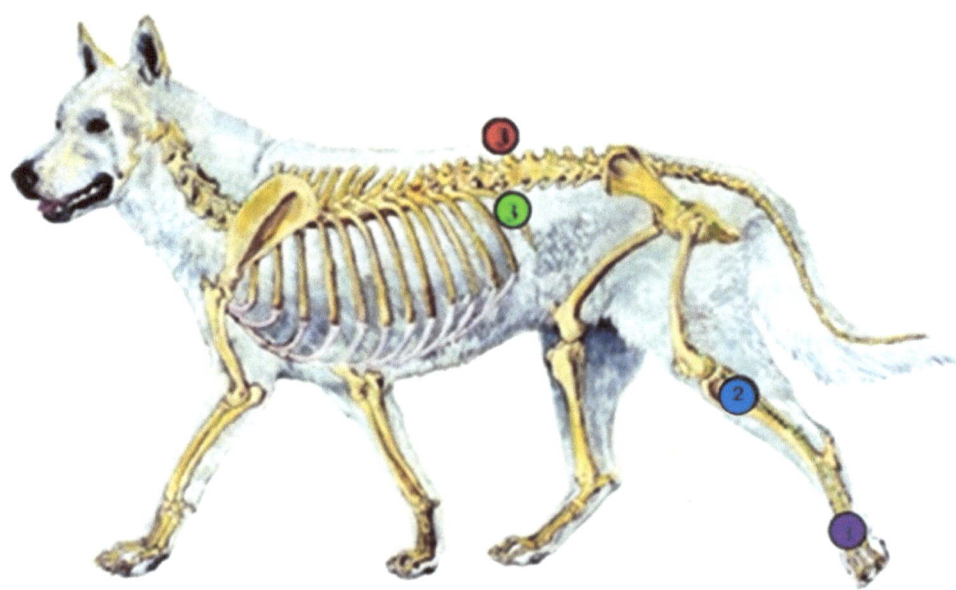

Signs: lack of motivation or drive, sleep pattern changes, extrcdeme chronic fatigue, salt craving, hair loss, dizziness.

Location	Indications	Color

1.	**Lv3** L&R outside hindleg between paw bones 2&3 at the joint	Liver & GB issues, endocrine & metabolic disorders (DM), hock pain & toxin removal	L-Violet R-Yellow
2.	**St36** L&R 1FW↓knee joint hind legs	Stomach, ulcers, constipation, diarrhea, weakness. Not for PG	L-Blue R-Orange
3.	**Bl22** 3FW each side of L1	Nephritis, hormonal imbalances, edema, disc issues.	L-Green R-Red

General Indications: Over/Underactive Adrenal glands, chronic fatigue, Insomnia, Hypoglycemia,

Directions: Shine colored light 15-20 seconds per point.

Allergies, Skin (LuLI)

If your pet start scratching, then chewing incessantly on one area a hot sore spot will almost immediately develop. Flea bites are one of the biggest culprits. But, over a period of time, if the pet continues to chew on himself, in spite of all that you have done to eradicate the fleas, he will develop a skin allergy, which is nothing more than just a very low intolerance to anything that comes in contact with his skin. The vets will shoot your pet full of steroids to stop the scratching and chewing, but this only helps temporarily and is not beneficial to your pet's long-term health. The main problem is breaking the "habit of chewing on himself". An oatmeal shampoo 2 times a week may help break the cycle as well as provide relief from itching. Daily color used on the areas listed above is another big help. Basically, anything you can do to break the habit will improve your pet's response.

Sarcoptic and Didactic mange are difficult to treat because they occur when the allergens have already lowered the immune response. This is another reason to treat any skin eruptions early. My experience with our very loving rescue dog, Wolfie was very sad indeed. He had been chained up by a previous owner, but Wolf broke free and got lost. The chain became embedded in his skin and had to be surgically removed when he was found and sent to the shelter. Unfortunately, just that physical trauma was enough to lower his resistance to skin infections. When we got him, he made it through the first winter with a full coat but when spring came he continued to shed until he was almost bald and the treatments by the vet were ineffective. Due to his old age and condition we had to make a difficult decision. This is why it is essential to catch any hot spots early and rebalance the meridians, which will be discussed in Section III.

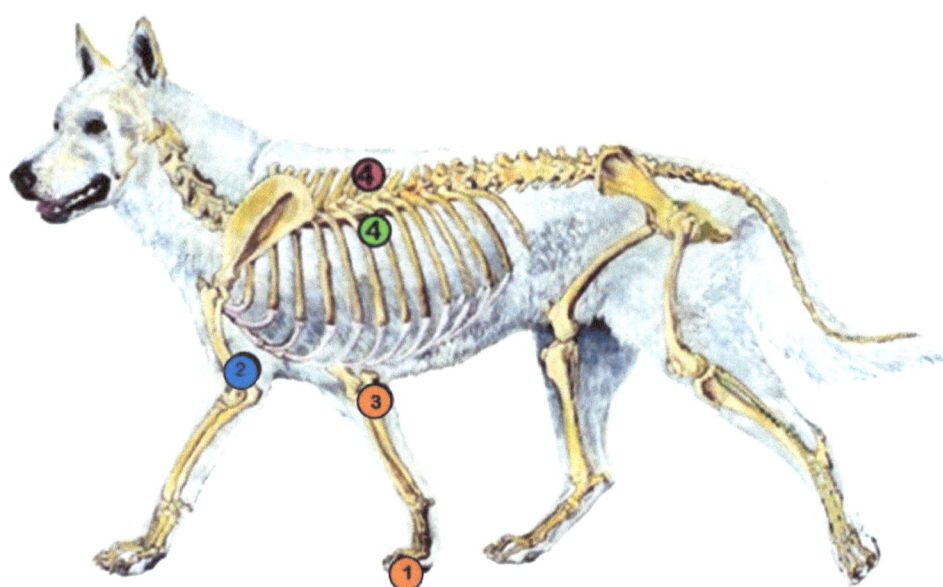

Signs: incessant scratching, Fur uneven or unclean, Red Inflamed Itchy Hot Spots, Loss of Fur or Dander, Brittle Dry Dull Coat, Fleas, Ticks, Blisters, Raised Rash, Scabs

	Location	Indications	Color
1.	**LI4** L&R inside forepaw in web between dewclaw & toe 1	Immune mediated skin issues. Sore throat, Cough, Neck, Shoulder pain, Lameness, Fever. Not for PG	L-Blue R-Orange

2.	**LI11** L&R front leg at joint where outside front leg meets body	Skin disorders, allergy, fever, endocrine, elbow & foreleg issues	L-Blue R-Orange
3.	**Lu5** L&R front leg at joint where inside front leg meets body	Immune-mediated skin disorders, fever, n/v, diarrhea, shoulder & elbow pain.	L-Blue R-Orange
4.	**Bl17** 3FW L&R of T7	Nonresponsive skin disorders, fever, blood disorders	L-Green R-Red

General Indications: For skin allergies, mange, hot spots, insect bites, burns.

Directions: Shine colored light 15-20 seconds per point.

- **Flea & Tick Repellant oils** are-- Palo Santo, Rosemary, Orange, Cedarwood, & Lemon.

- **Essential Oils for treating skin allergies and breaking the cycle** —Eucalyptus, Cedarwood, Geranium, Helichrysum, Naouli, and German Chamomile. Also, Melaleuca or Tea Tree oil applied on the affected areas will heal up sore spots.

Anger & Aggression (LvGB)

Anger or Aggression is the predominant emotion of the Liver/Gall Bladder Meridians. Negative emotions form blockages in the meridian pathways leading to physical disease.

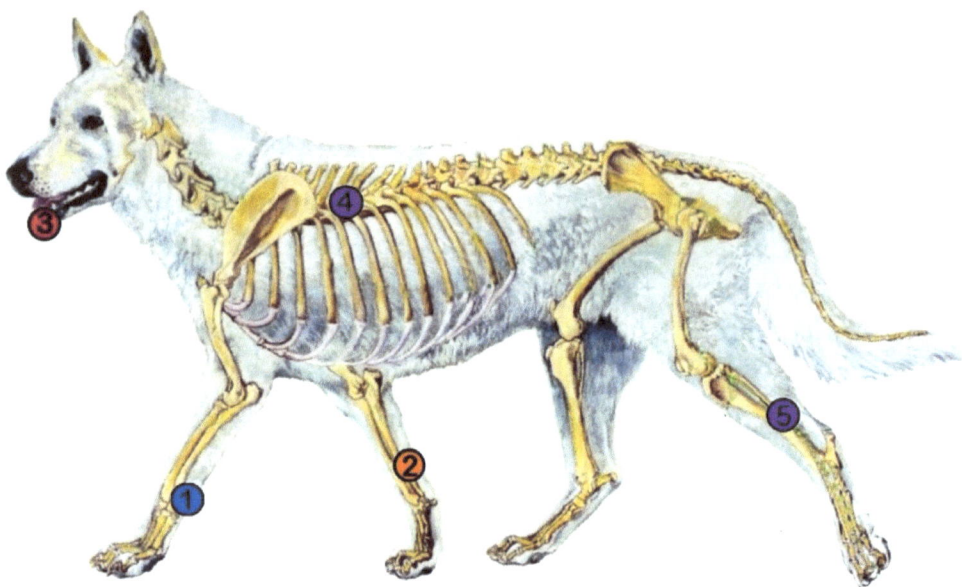

Signs: growls, bites, fights, dominates, fear, apprehension

	Location	Indications	Color
1.	**Ht7** L&R outside frontleg at wrist joint	Anxiety, fever, anorexia, epilepsy, behavior issues	L-Blue R-Orange
2.	**Pc5** L&R inside frontleg 4FW↑ elbow joint	Seizures, severe agitation, n/v, palpitations	L-Blue R-Orange
3.	**CV24** center lower lip	Behavioral disorders, mania, seizures, gingivitis, gum or tooth pain	Red
4.	**GV11** in IC space T5-6	aggression	Violet
5.	**St40** L&R outside hindleg 3FW↑elbow joint	Depression, mania, anxiety, hind limb paralysis, GI disorders	L-Violet R-Yellow

<u>General Indications</u>: For aggressive behavior issues around other animals as well as people.

<u>Directions</u>: Shine colored light 15-20 seconds per point.

💧 **Essential oils**—Roman Chamomile, Valerian Root, & Lavender help to calm and soothe aggression and agitation.

Anxiety (KiBl)

Anxiety or **Worry** is the predominant emotion of the Stomach/Spleen Meridians. Negative emotions form blockages in the meridian pathways leading to physical disease.

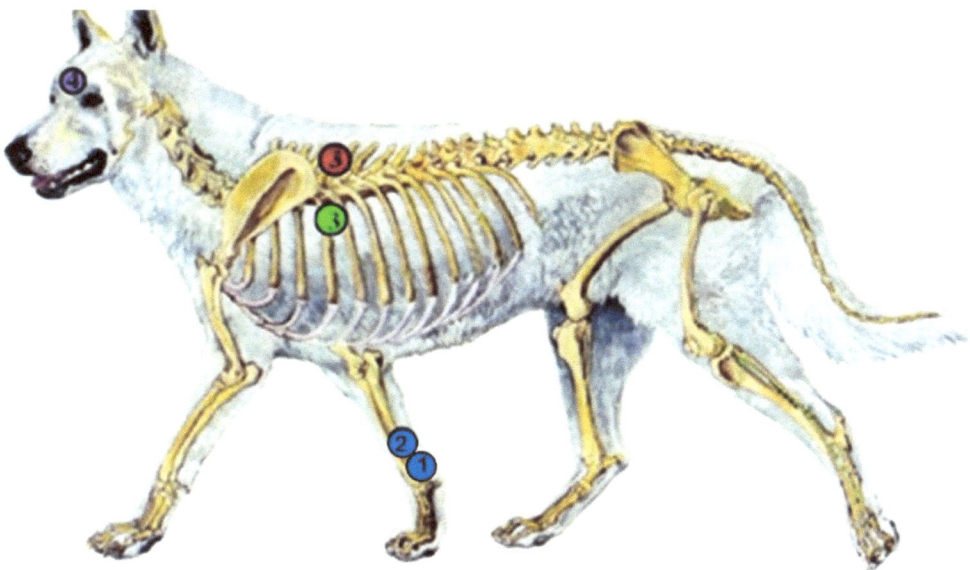

Signs: compulsive, marking territory, destructive tendencies

	Location	Indications	Color
1.	**Pc6**- L&R 4FW↑joint on inside of front leg	Seizures, agitation, n/v, palpitations	L-Turquoise R- Orange
2.	**Pc7**-L&R just ↑joint on inside of front leg	Epilepsy, fever, anxiety, n/v.	L-Turquoise R- Orange
3.	**Bl15** 3FW L&R of T5	Disorientation, calms, seizures, chest pain	L-Green R-Red
4.	**Yin Trang** – Pineal gland. Between eyebrows	Sleep and Melatonin production, anxiety	Violet

General Indications: For anxiousness, agitation, confusion, epilepsy, confusion

Directions: Shine colored light 15-20 seconds per point.

💧 Essential oils—Roman Chamomile, Valerian Root, & Lavender help to calm and soothe anxiety.

Arthritis (SpSt)

Arthritis, once it has begun its degenerative process is very difficult to treat. Thus, that is why there is a multitude of acupoints. If your pet won't hold still long enough for this full treatment, try treating just the points directed on the areas of most concern, such as GB29 for hip joints.

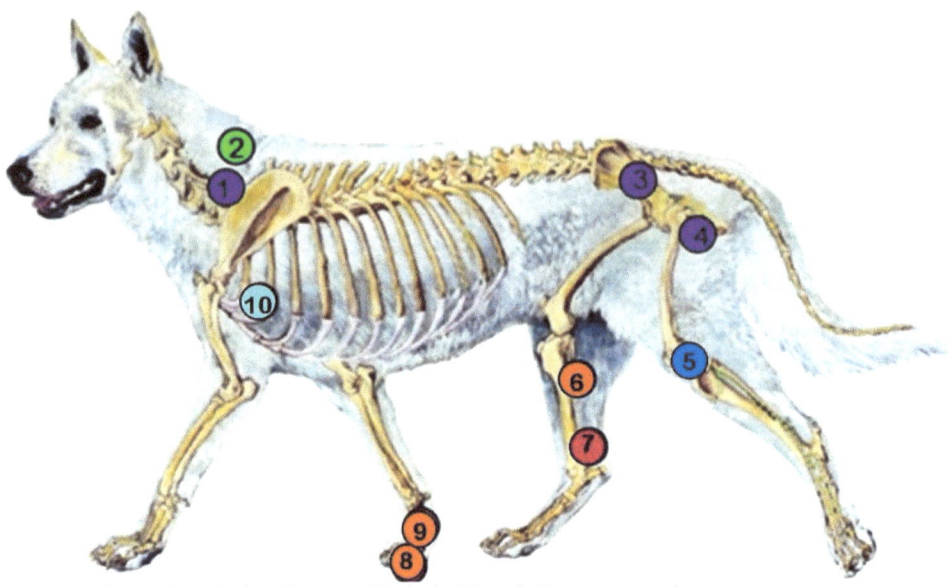

Signs: stiffness & pain in joints, particularly hips, fatigue, anorexia.

	Location	Indications	Color
1.	**GV14** between C7 &T1 on spine	Fever, cough, cervical pain, spondylosis, immune system.	Violet
2.	**Bl11** 3FW L&R end of cervical spine	Osteoarthritis, cervical, thoracic & disc disease & joint pain	L-Green R-Red
3.	**GB29** 3FW L&R on coccyx where it meets tail	LBP, hip joint issues, osteoarthritis	L-Violet R-Yellow
4.	**GB33** L&R hip joint hindleg	Stifle pain & osteoarthritis	L- Violet R- Yellow
5.	**St35** L&R outside knee joint of hindleg.	stifle pain & inflammation, osteoarthritis, lower limb weakness	L-Blue R-Orange
6.	**Sp9** L&R inside hindleg ↓ hip joint in depression above calf muscle.	Incontinence, stifle pain, edema	L-Blue R-Orange
7.	**K3** L&R 1FW↑ inside hindleg hock	Arthritis, local swelling of hock, LBP, Kidney, ear issues	L-Green R-Red
8.	**LI4** L&R inside forepaw in web between dewclaw & toe 1	Immune mediated skin issues. Sore throat, Cough, Neck, Shoulder pain, Lameness, Fever. Not for PG	L-Blue R-Orange

9.	**TH3** L&R inside front paw 1FW↑joint	Eye & ear issues, fever, shoulder pain	L-Turquoise R- Orange
10	**SI9** L&R at end of 2nd rib on front shoulder joint	Pain, stiffness, paralysis, arthritis of scapula, shoulder, neck & forearm. Inflammation	L-Turquoise R- Orange

General Indications: For arthritis and all joint & vertebrae pain & disease.

Directions: Shine colored light 15-20 seconds per point.

Bladder / Urinary Issues (KiBl)

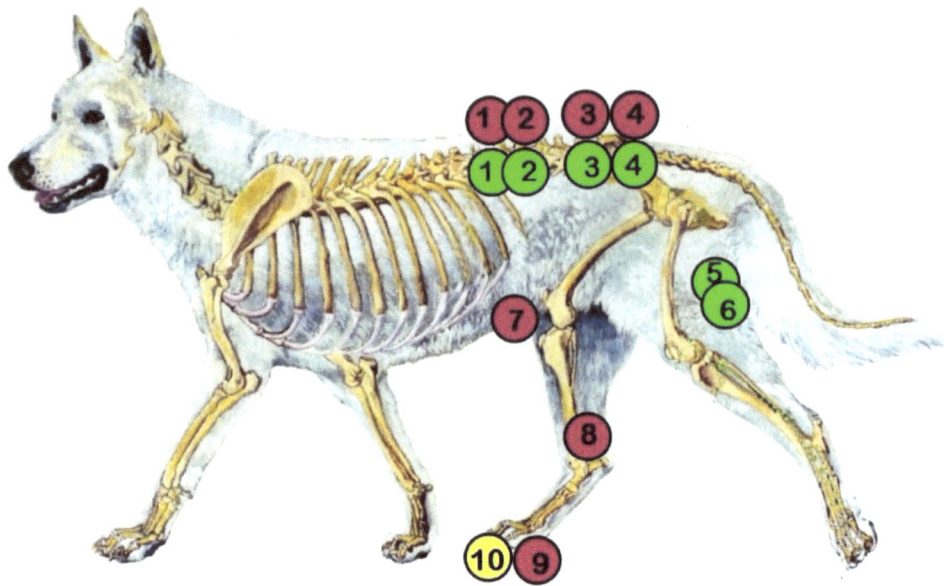

Signs: n/v, passing only small amounts of urine; swelling ankles; fatigue; loss of appetite; ↑BP; itchy; ammonia odor of breathe; mouth ulcers; tongue inflammation

	Location	Indications	Color
1.	**Bl22** 3FW each side of L1	Chronic kidney/bladder issues, hormonal imbalances, edema, spinal issues.	L-Green R-Red
2.	**Bl23** 3FW each side of L2	Weakness, seizures, ears, eyes, LBP, kidney, focus, brain	L-Green R-Red
3.	**Bl26** 3FW each side of L6	Incontinence, LBP, sciatica, constipation, diarrhea, impotence	L-Green R-Red
4.	**Bl28** 3FW each side of 2nd hole on sacrum before iliac crest	Urinary issues, constipation, diarrhea, spinal pain	L-Green R-Red
5.	**Bl39** 1FW↑ L&R of Bl40	Incontinence, edema, hock pain, kidney pain, LBP	L-Green R-Red
6.	**Bl40** L&R on outside & backside of hindleg where it meets body.	LBP, Hips, Stifles, incontinence, AI disorders, spondylosis, paralysis	L-Green R-Red
7.	**CV3** 5FW ↓from navel	Incontinence, renal issues, infertility	Red or IR
8.	**Ki3** L&R inside hindleg 1FW↑elbow joint.	Kidney issues & renal failure, arthritis, hock swelling, LBP, ears, PMS	L-Green R-Red
9.	**Ki1** L&R inside hindleg on 1st toe of paw	Incontinence, infertility, heatstroke, fever	L-Green R-Red
10.	**Lv2** L&R inside hindleg on 2nd toe of paw	Eye, PMS, incontinence or retention, epilepsy	L- Violet R- Yellow

General Indications: For all Kidney/Bladder disorders—incontinence or retention, pain, kidney failure.

Directions: Shine colored light 15-20 seconds per point.

Cancer (HtSl)

Cancer cells grow at a faster rate than normal healthy cells. The color Red stimulates cell growth and repair while it reduces inflammation and pain; so it would not be suitable for use on cancer cells. With Cancer, you have to get the immune system to recognize cancer cells as foreign cells. The longer the cancer cells are allowed to become part of the body, the less likely the body is to recognize them as foreign. This is where it is important to assess your pet's health on a regular basis and do the immune regulatory treatment 1st on a daily basis.

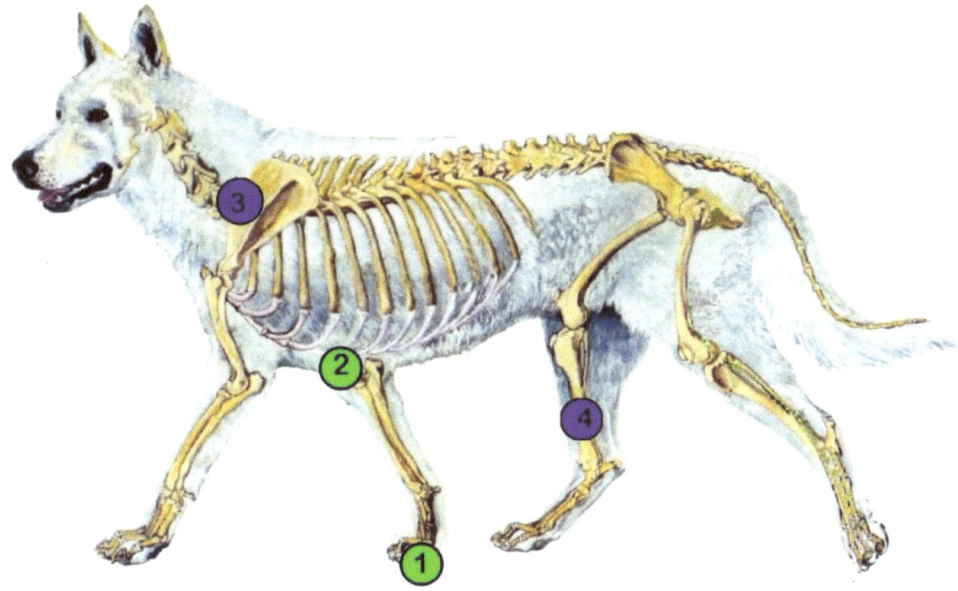

Signs: visible tumors, warts, tenderness to touch, sad, dull eyes, not eating

	Location	Indications	Color
1.	**LI4** L&R inside forepaw in web between dewclaw & toe 1	Immune mediated skin issues. Sore throat, Cough, Neck, Shoulder pain, Lameness, Fever. Not for PG	Green
2.	**Lu5** L&R front leg at joint where inside front leg meets body	Immune-mediated skin disorders, fever, n/v, diarrhea, shoulder & elbow pain.	Green
3.	**GV14** between C7 &T1 on spine	Fever, cough, cervical pain, spondylosis, immune system.	Violet
4.	**Sp6** L&R inside hindleg 3FW↑ hock	Hypothyroidism, edema, fatigue, incontinence, immune, not for PG	Violet

General Indications: For skin cancers, tumors, warts, and other cancers

Directions: Shine colored light 15-20 seconds per point.

- **Essential oils**—Frankincense is as good as you get for cancer. Find a good quality oil though. Prices for a 15ml bottle range from $35-$100. If you go through an MLM like DoTerra or Young Living you will pay more than if you find an independent wholesaler like Liberty Natural Oils. One thing I like about Liberty is that they publish their MSDS (material safety data sheets) which list where the oils come from, their purity, whether they are safe for oral consumption or just for topical application.

Confusion (LvGB)

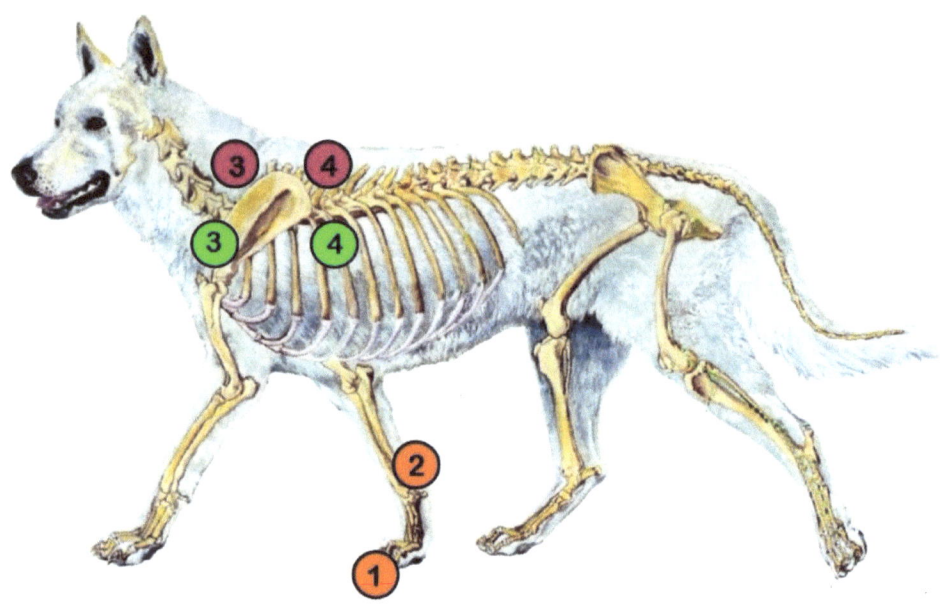

Signs: disorientation to person, place or thing; lack of self-confidence; unfocused, untidy, unrestful.

	Location	Indications	Color
1.	**Pc9** L&R inside frontleg at nailbed, 3rd digit	Confusion, shock, LOC, heatstroke, fever	L-Turquoise R- Orange
2.	**Pc5** L&R inside frontleg 4FW from elbow.	Confusion, seizures, agitation, n/v, chest pain.	L-Turquoise R- Orange
3.	**Ki27** L&R between sternum & 1st rib	Disorientation, anxiety, n/v, anorexia, asthma, cough, chest pain	L-Green R-Red
4.	**Bl15** 3FW L&R of T5	Disorientation, calms, seizures, chest pain	L-Green R-Red

General Indications: For inability to focus on current setting, instability of mood; uncleanliness.

Directions: Shine colored light 15-20 seconds per point.

Constipation (SpSt)

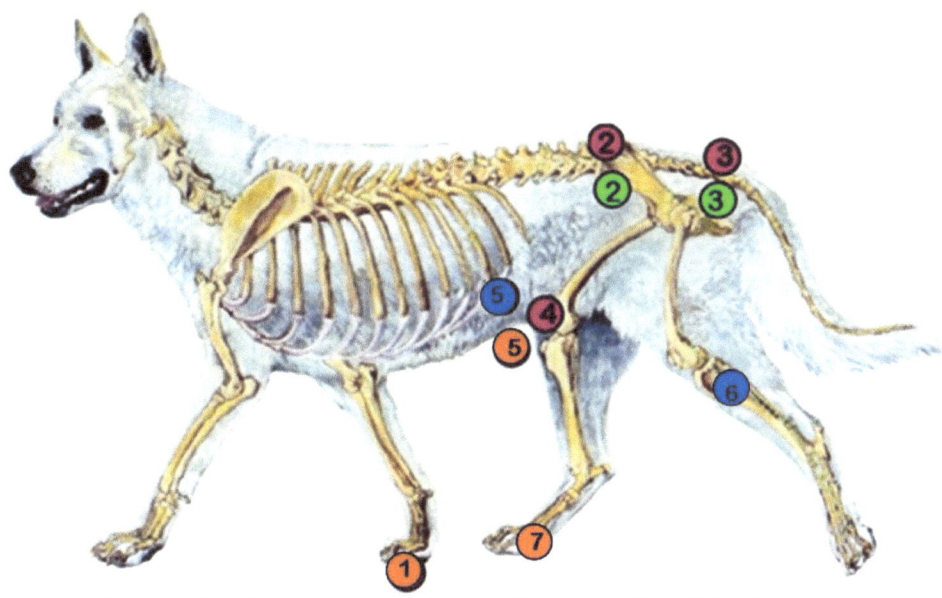

Signs: Infrequent BM, loss of appetite, dehydration, abdominal distention

	Location	Indications	Color
1.	**LI4** L&R inside forepaw in web between dewclaw & toe 1	Immune mediated skin issues. Sore throat, Cough, Neck, Shoulder pain, Lameness, Fever. Not for PG	L-Blue R-Orange
2.	**Bl26** 3FW each side of L6	Incontinence, LBP, sciatica, constipation, diarrhea, impotence	L-Green R-Red
3.	**Bl28** 3FW each side of Sacrum	Urinary issues, constipation & diarrhea, spinal pain	L-Green R-Red
4.	**CV6** 2FW↓ navel	Chronic diarrhea, weakness, constipation, abdominal pain	Red or IR
5.	**St25** 3FW each side of navel	GI disorders, abdominal masses, diarrhea or constipation, n/v	L-Blue R-Orange
6.	**St36** L&R 1FW↓knee joint hind legs	Stomach, ulcers, constipation, diarrhea, weakness. Not for PG	L-Blue R-Orange
7.	**Sp3** L&R on inside hindleg 2FW↑paw joint	Diarrhea, constipation, digestion, obesity	L-Blue R-Orange

General Indications: For difficultly passing hard stool and infrequent BM, ↓peristalsis & low motility.

Directions: Shine colored light 15-20 seconds per point. Green color acts as a laxative and can be used on both sides of the body instead of its complementary color-Red. Complementary colors are used for balancing the body side to side.

💧 Peppermint essential oil is good for gas cramps and bloating that typically accompanies constipation.

Depression (LuLI)

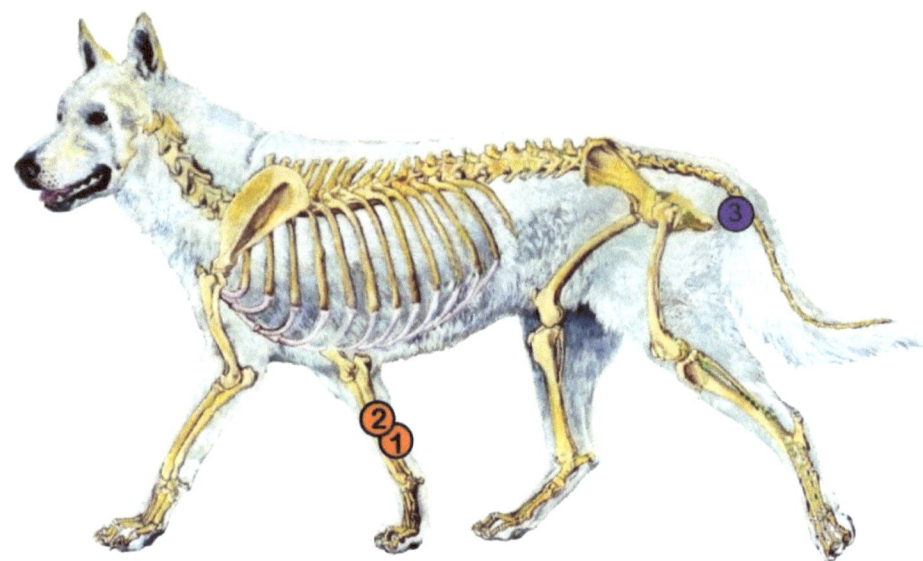

Signs: fatigue, lack of motivation, sleeps a lot, anorexia

	Location	Indications	Color
1.	**Pc5** L&R inside frontleg 4FW↑ elbow joint	Seizures, severe agitation, n/v, palpitations	L-Turquoise R- Orange
2.	**Pc6**- L&R 5FW↑joint on inside of front leg	Seizures, agitation, n/v, palpitations	L-Turquoise R- Orange
3.	**GV1** midline just under the tail	Spinal stiffness, LBP, seizures, diarrhea, constipation, depression, fatigue	Violet

General Indications: For Lung/Large Intestine issues, melancholy, depression, sadness, seizures, agitation

Directions: Shine colored light 15-20 seconds per point.

Orange on underside of back paw. Indigo on top of back paw.

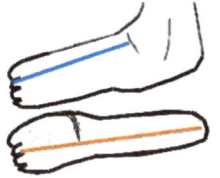

Diabetes (SpSt)

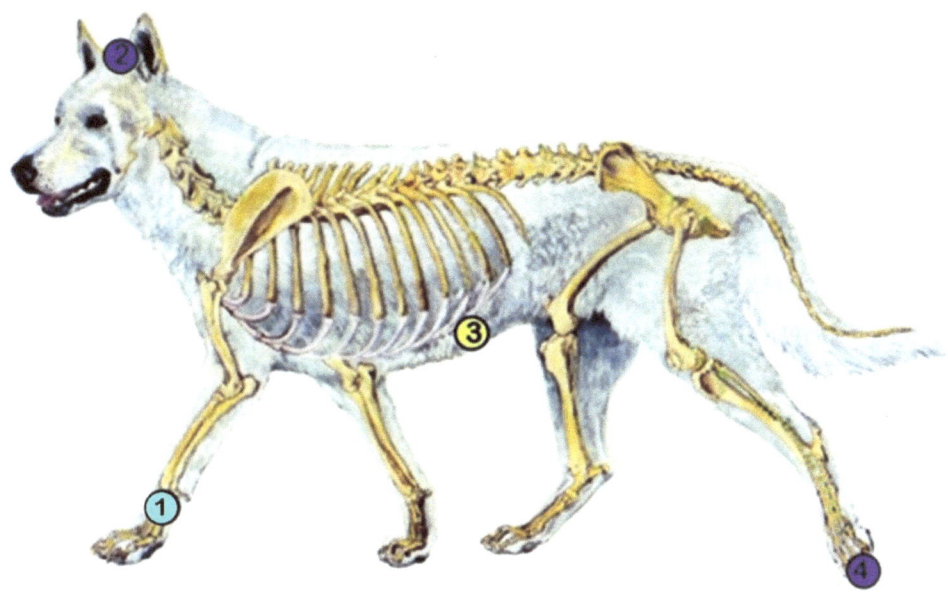

Signs: excessive urination and/or thirst; hunger, weight change, anorexia, lethargy, depression; n/v

	Location	Indications	Color
1.	**TH4** L&R outside frontleg just ↓elbow	Fatigue, swelling & pain of front paw & shoulder, Diabetes	L-Turquoise R- Orange
2.	**GV20** top head; ↑ from top of ears	Pituitary issues, Diabetes, neck stiffness, insomnia, shock, seizures	Violet
3.	**CV12** midway from xyphoid to navel	Pancreas, Diabetes, weakness, urine retention, infertility.	Yellow
4.	**Lv3** L&R outside hindleg between paw bones 2&3 at the joint	Liver & GB issues, endocrine & metabolic disorders (DM), hock pain & toxin removal	L- Violet R- Yellow

General Indications: For Endocrine, Pancreatic & Metabolic disorders—Diabetes, Pancreatitis, Liver & GB issues.

Directions: Shine colored light 15-20 seconds per point.

Diarrhea (LuLI)

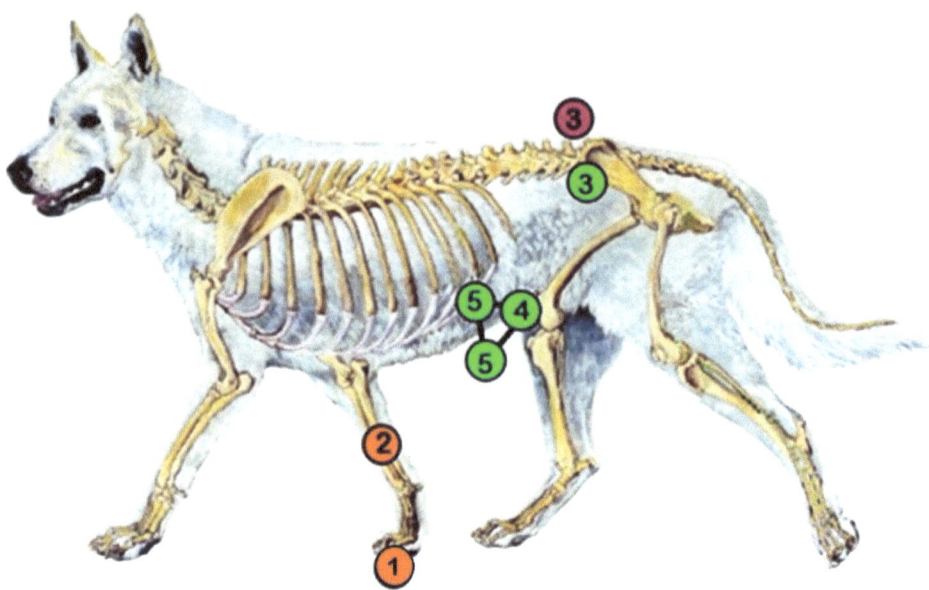

Signs: Frequent watery stool with or without mucous

	Location	Indications	Color
1.	**LI4** L&R inside forepaw in web between dewclaw & toe 1	Immune mediated skin issues. Sore throat, Cough, Neck, Shoulder pain, Lameness, Fever. Not for PG	L-Blue R-Orange
2.	**Pc6**- L&R 4FW↑joint on inside of front leg	Seizures, agitation, n/v, palpitations	L-Turquoise R- Orange
3.	**Bl26** 3FW each side of L6	Incontinence, LBP, sciatica, constipation, diarrhea, impotence	L-Green R-Red
4.	**CV6** 2FW↓ navel	Chronic diarrhea, weakness, constipation, abdominal pain	Green
5.	**St25** 3FW each side of navel	GI disorders, abdominal masses, diarrhea or constipation, n/v	L- Green R- Green

General Indications: For acute or chronic diarrhea and other GI disorders

Directions: Shine colored light 15-20 seconds per point. Please note that points 4 & 5 are **all** in Green. The color green cools and neutralizes GI infection and discomfort. The 3-point triangle also has a calming effect upon the entire abdominal region.

Ear Disorders (KiBl)

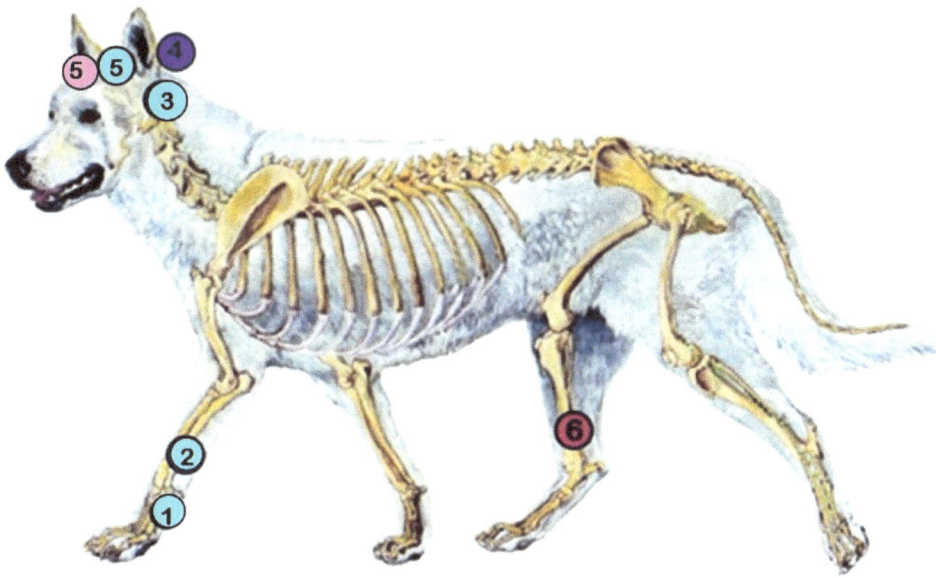

Signs: Scratching, shaking head, odor, dark debris or blood, dizziness, balance issues, unresponsive to loud or soft noises nearby.

	Location	Indications	Color
1.	**Th3** L&R outside frontleg 2FW↑ wrist joint	Ear & Eye disorders, fever, shoulder pain, local joint pain	L-Turquoise R- Orange
2.	**TH5** L&R outside frontleg 2FW↑ elbow joint	Otitis, conjunctivitis, fever, shoulder & neck pain, lameness	L-Turquoise R- Orange
3.	**TH17** L&R 2FW ↓bottom of ears	Ear disorders, seizures, TMJ& neck pain	L-Turquoise R- Orange
4.	**GV16** back crown of head or end of occiput	Epilepsy, stroke, eye vision, hearing DDD	Violet or UV
5.	**SI19** L&R at bottom of ear where it meets forehead	Deafness & ear problems, otitis, seizures	L Turquoise R Pink *
6.	**K3** L&R inside hindleg 1FW↑hock joint.	Kidney issues & renal failure, arthritis, hock swelling, LBP, ears, PMS	L-Green R-Red

General Indications: For acute or chronic ear infections, earaches, deafness, dizziness, or Kidney/Bladder issues.

Directions: Shine colored light 15-20 seconds per point.

💧 **Essential oils**—Bergamot and Geranium. Basil helps with earache pain.

Epilepsy (HtSI)

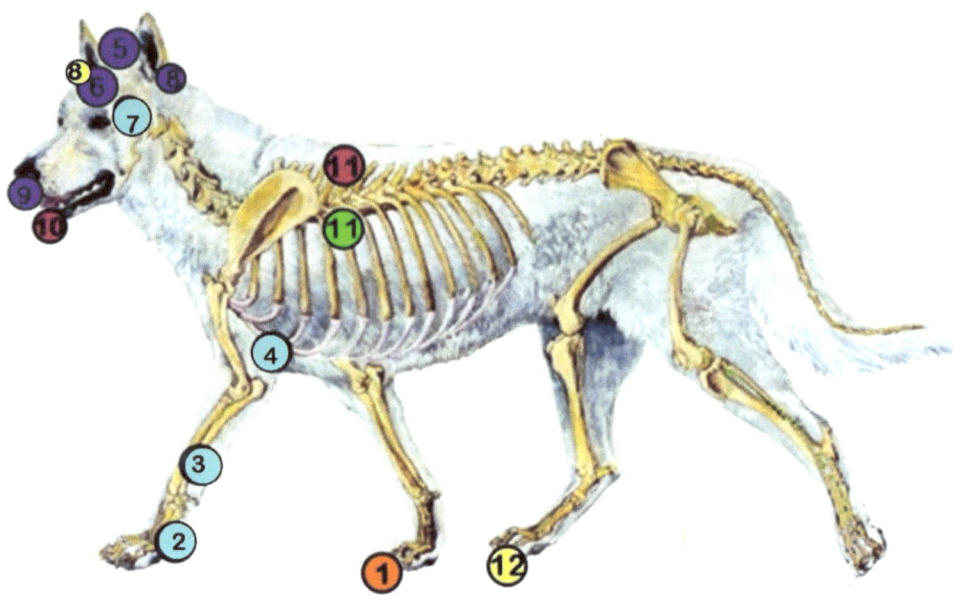

Signs: petit mal or grand mal seizures, head shakes, pupil dilation, weakness, drooling, foaming of mouth

	Location	Indications	Color
1.	**Pc9** L&R inside frontleg, 3rd toe at nailbed	Fever, heatstroke, shock, LOC	L- Turquoise R- Orange
2.	**SI3** L&R Outside frontleg wrist joint	Fever, conjunctivitis, neck & shoulder pain, epilepsy.	L Turquoise R Pink *
3.	**SI5** L&R Outside frontleg 2FW↑ elbow joint	Seizures, fear, tinnitus, fever.	L Turquoise R Pink *
4.	**SI8** Outside frontleg where leg meets body	Elbow pain, seizures, neck, shoulder & teeth pain.	L Turquoise R Pink *
5.	**GV20** top head; ↑ from top of ears	Pituitary issues, Diabetes, neck stiffness, insomnia, shock, seizures	Violet
6.	**GV21** front edge of ears	Epilepsy, ADHD	Violet
7.	**TH23** L&R end of eyebrow in hole	Epilepsy, eye disorders, dental issues, facial paralysis	L- Turquoise R- Orange
8.	**GB20** bottom base of ear	Epilepsy, eye & neck issues	L- Violet R- Yellow
9.	**GV26** mid upper lip	Shock, heatstroke, coma, seizures, spinal pain	Violet
10.	**CV24** center lower lip	Behavioral disorders, mania, seizures, gingivitis, gum or tooth pain	Red or IR
11.	**BI15** 3FW L&R of T5	Disorientation, calms, seizures, chest pain	L- Green R- Red
12.	**Lv2** L&R inside hindleg on 2nd toe of paw	Eye, PMS, incontinence or retention, epilepsy	L- Violet R- Yellow

General Indications: For convulsions, either grand mal or petit mal seizures, loss of consciousness, shock, heat stroke. **Directions**: Shine colored light 15-20 seconds per point.

Eye disorders (LvGB)

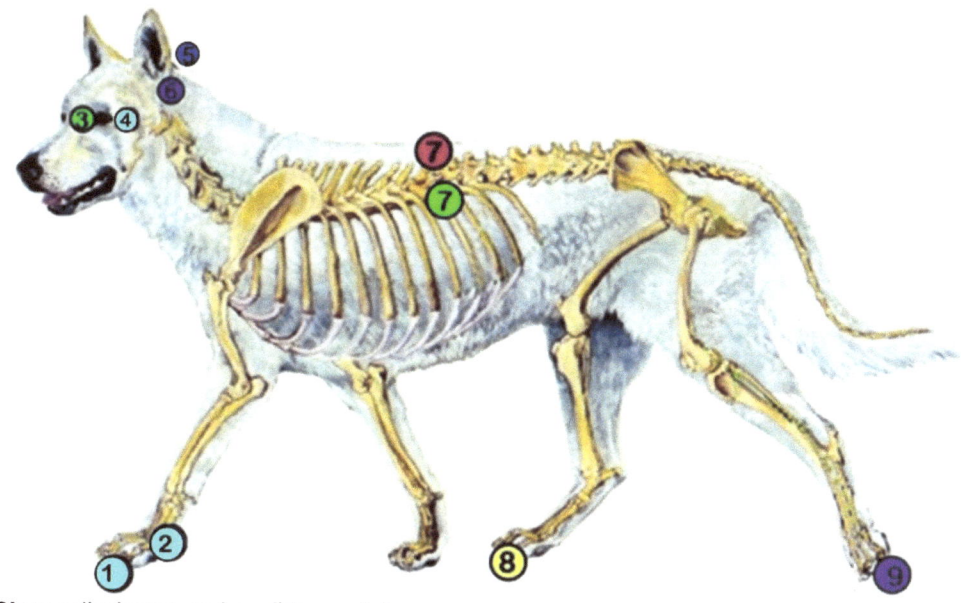

Signs: discharge, red eyelids, squinting

	Location	Indications	Color
1.	TH1 L&R outside front paw at 4th nailbed	Fever, conjunctivitis, deafness, tinnitus, shoulder pain	L Turquoise R Pink *
2.	TH3 L&R outside front paw at wrist joint	Ear & eye disorders, fever, shoulder pain, local joint pain	L Turquoise R Pink *
3.	Bl1 L&R inner eye corners	All eye issues, uveitis, conjunctivitis, myopia, optic nerve atrophy.	L-Green R-Red
4.	TH23 L&R end of eyebrow in hole	Epilepsy, eye disorders, dental issues, facial paralysis	L Turquoise R Pink *
5.	GV16 back crown of head or end of occiput	Epilepsy, stroke, eye vision, hearing DDD	Violet or UV
6.	GB20 bottom base of ear	Epilepsy, eye & neck issues	L- Violet R- Yellow
7.	Bl18 3FW L&R T10	Liver/GB or any eye issues, seizures, chronic fatigue.	L-Green R-Red
8.	Lv2 L&R inside hindleg on 2nd toe of paw	Eye, PMS, incontinence or retention, epilepsy	L- Violet R- Yellow
9.	GB44 L&R outside paw of hindleg at 4thnailbed	Fever, hypertension, shock, eye issues	L- Violet R- Yellow

General Indications: For eye infections, eye disorders, Liver/GB issues

Directions: Shine colored light 15-20 seconds per point.

Fear (KiBl)

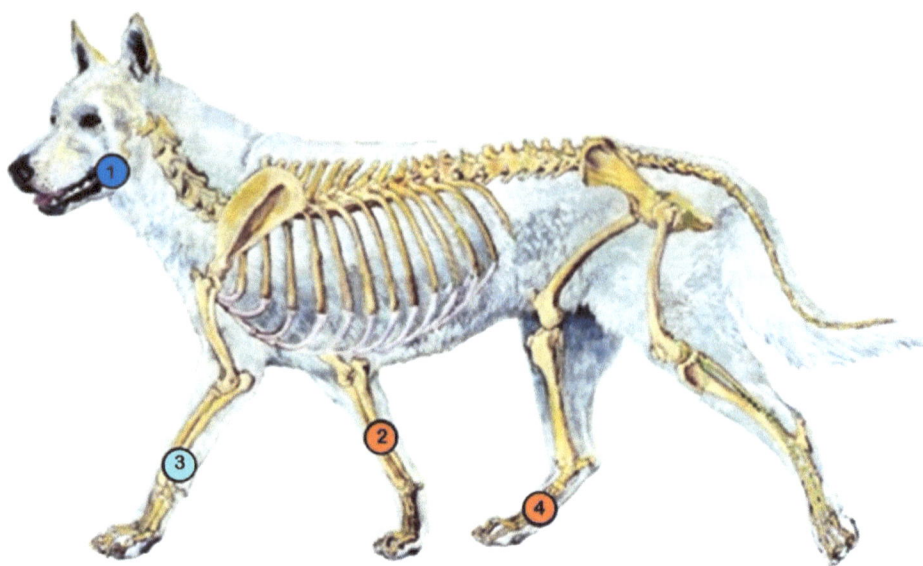

Signs: hiding out, growling or hissing, biting

	Location	Indications	Color
1.	**St4** L&R on cheek	Fear, anger, jaw tension, facial paralysis	L-Blue R-Orange
2.	**Pc4** L&R inside front leg 3FW↑wrist joint	Calms during a fearful situation	L-Turquoise R- Orange
3.	**Sl5** L&R Outside frontleg 2FW↑ elbow joint	Seizures, fear, tinnitus, fever.	L Turquoise R Pink *
4.	**Sp3** L&R on inside hindleg 2FW↑paw joint	Diarrhea, constipation, digestion, obesity	L-Blue R-Orange

General Indications: For fearful behavior and other kidney/bladder issues.

Directions: Shine colored light 15-20 seconds per point.

💧 **Essential oils**—Roman Chamomile, Valerian Root, & Lavender help to calm fear.

Fever (HtSI)

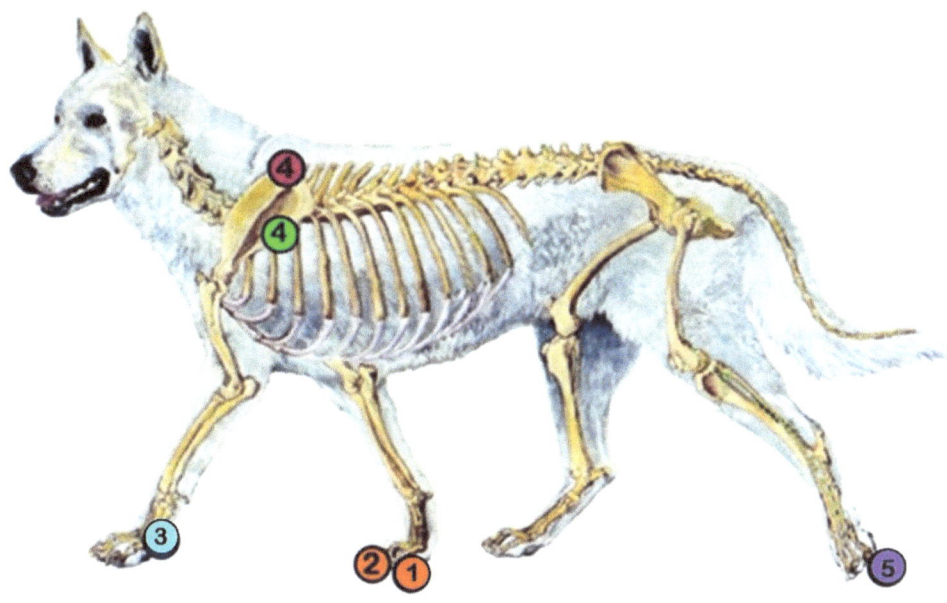

Signs: rectal temperature ↑; fatigue, weakness, shivering, anorexia, ↑HR ↑RR

	Location	Indications	Color
1.	**LI4** L&R inside forepaw in web between dewclaw & toe 1	Immune mediated skin issues. Sore throat, Cough, Neck, Shoulder pain, Lameness, Fever. Not for PG	L-Blue R-Orange
2.	**Pc9** L&R inside frontleg, 3rd toe at nailbed	Fever, heatstroke, shock, LOC	L-Turquoise R- Orange
3.	**TH3** L&R outside front paw at wrist joint	Ear & eye disorders, fever, shoulder pain, local joint pain	L-Turquoise R- Orange
4.	**Bl12** 3FWL&R T2	Neck & chest pain, nasal congestion, fever	L-Green R-Red
5.	**GB44** L&R outside paw of hindleg at 4th nailbed	Fever, hypertension, shock, eye issues	L- Violet R- Yellow

General Indications: For high fever, heatstroke

Directions: Shine colored light 15-20 seconds per point.

Gastrointestinal Disorders (SpSt)

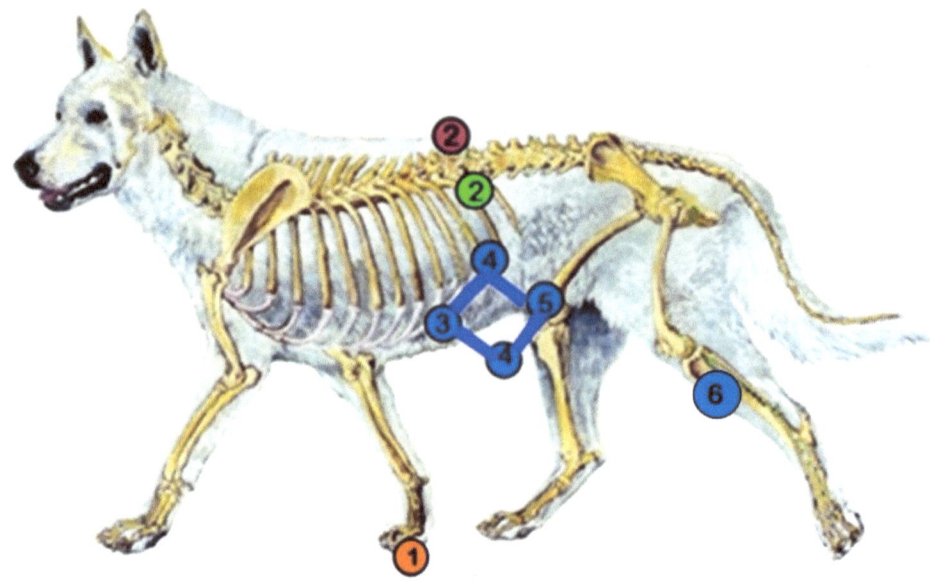

Signs: Vomiting, weight loss, hot ears or nose, stiff, weak hind legs.

	Location	Indications	Color
1.	**LI4** L&R inside forepaw in web between dewclaw & toe 1	Immune mediated skin issues. Sore throat, Cough, Neck, Shoulder pain, Lameness, Fever. Not for PG	L-Blue R-Orange
2.	**Bl21** 3FW each side of T13	GI issues, edema, diarrhea, weakness, n/v, LBP	L-Green R-Red
3.	**CV12** midway from xyphoid to navel	Pancreas, Diabetes, weakness, urine retention, infertility.	Blue
4.	**Lv13** L&R at lowest point 12th rib on sides	Food stagnation, abdominal masses & pain, fatigue, liver & stomach issues	Blue
5.	**CV8** on navel	Chronic diarrhea, weakness, constipation, abdominal pain	Blue
6.	**St36** L&R 1FW↓knee joint hind legs	Stomach, ulcers, constipation, diarrhea, weakness. Not for PG	L-Blue R-Orange

General Indications: For nausea/vomiting, diarrhea, abdominal pain, other GI issues.

Directions: Shine colored light 15-20 seconds per point. Points 3-5 are part of the Stomach Diamond which works amazingly well at relieving nausea and diarrhea. Put a few drops of peppermint oil on the point sites before color.

- Essential Oils—Peppermint & Ginger are great for stomachaches.

- For diarrhea also try Color Reflexology Orange on underside of back paw. Indigo on top of back paw. Stroke lines back & forth 30 seconds each on both back paws.

Heart-Lung Issues (HtSI)

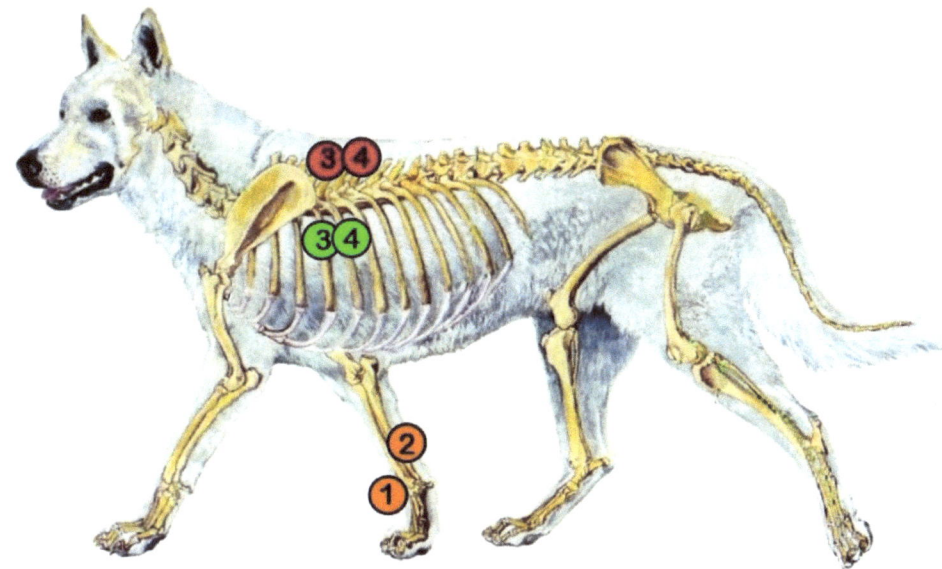

Signs: shortness of breath, wheezing, easily fatigued, weakness

	Location	Indications	Color
1.	**Pc3**- L&R inside frontleg crease of elbow	Heatstroke, fever, palpitations, shoulder & elbow pain, diarrhea	L-Turquoise R- Orange
2.	**Pc6**- L&R 4FW↑joint on inside of front leg	Seizures, agitation, n/v, palpitations	L-Turquoise R- Orange
3.	**Bl14** 3FW L&R of T4	Anxiety, palpitations, cough, heart irregularities	L-Green R-Red
4.	**Bl15** 3FW L&R of T5	Disorientation, calms, seizures, chest pain	L-Green R-Red

<u>**General Indications**</u>: For palpitations, fever, heatstroke and other Lung/Large Intestine or Heart/SI issues.

<u>**Directions**</u>: Shine colored light 15-20 seconds per point.

Heat Stroke (HtSl)

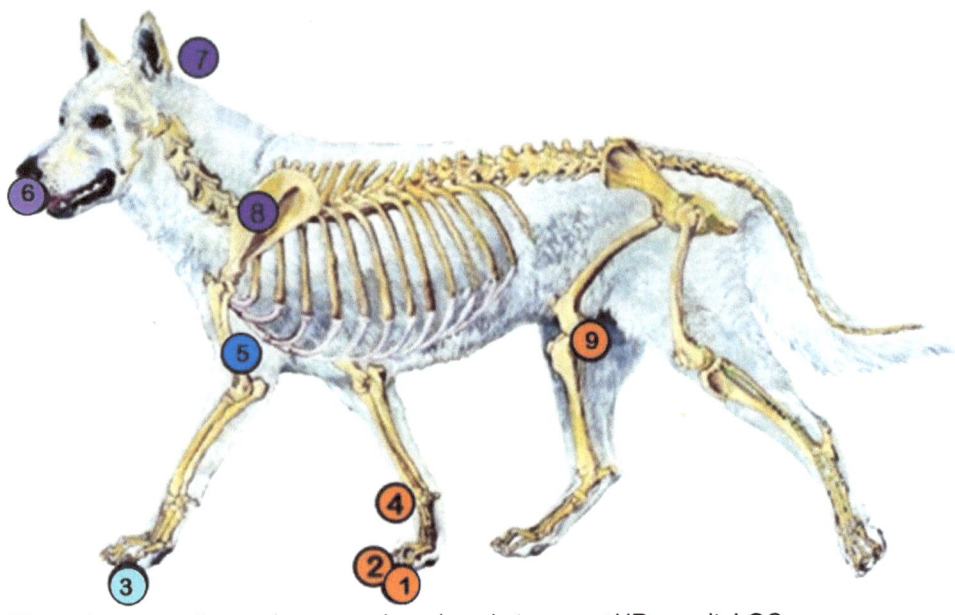

Signs: fever, panting, pale gums, cherry/purple tongue, ↑HR, vomit, LOC

	Location	Indications	Color
1.	**LI4** L&R inside forepaw in web between dewclaw & toe 1	Immune mediated skin issues. Sore throat, Cough, Neck, Shoulder pain, Lameness, Fever. Not for PG	L-Blue R-Orange
2.	**Pc9** L&R inside frontleg at nailbed, 3rd digit	Confusion, shock, LOC, heatstroke, fever	L-Turquoise R- Orange
3.	**SI1** L&R outside 5th toe front paws	Fever, coma, shoulder pain, lactations	L Turquoise R Pink *
4.	**Pc3-** L&R inside frontleg crease of elbow	Heatstroke, fever, palpitations, shoulder & elbow pain, diarrhea	L-Turquoise R- Orange
5.	**LI11** L&R front leg at joint where outside front leg meets body	Skin disorders, allergy, fever, endocrine, elbow & foreleg issues	L-Blue R-Orange
6.	**GV26** mid upper lip	Shock, heatstroke, coma, seizures, spinal pain	Violet
7.	**GV16** back crown of head or end of occiput	Epilepsy, stroke, eye vision, hearing DDD	Violet or UV
8.	**GV14** between C7 &T1 on spine	Fever, cough, cervical pain, spondylosis, immune system.	Violet
9.	**Sp10** L&R inside hindleg opposite hip where leg meets body	Blood deficiency, fever	L-Blue R-Orange

General Indications: For high fever & convulsion, shock, LOC.

Directions: Shine colored light 15-20 seconds per point.

Hip Dysplasia (SpSt)

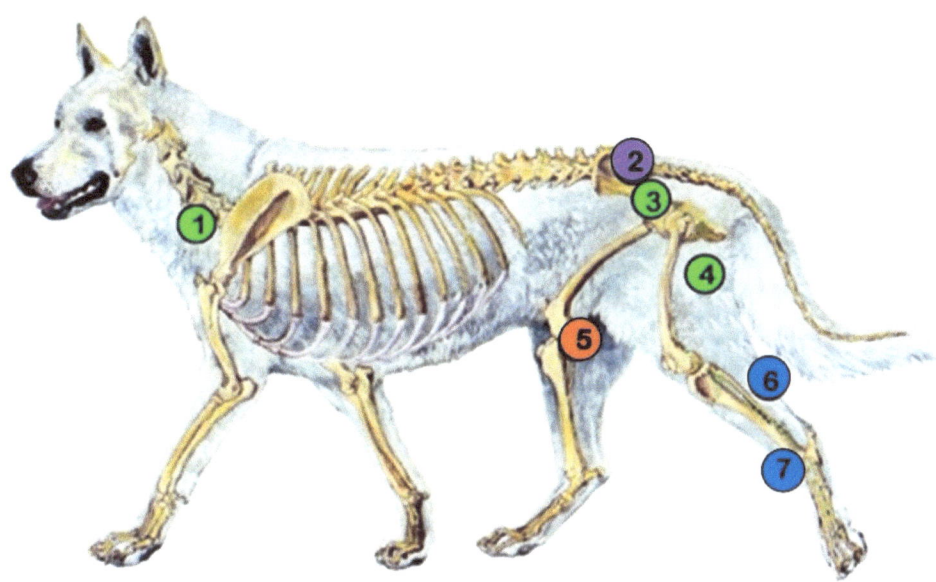

Signs: Lame, stiff, pain getting up & down, sensitive to touch

	Location	Indications	Color
1.	**Bl11** 3FW L&R end of cervical spine	Osteoarthritis, cervical, thoracic & disc disease & joint pain	L-Green R-Red
2.	**GB29** 3FW L&R on coccyx where it meets tail	LBP, hip joint issues, osteoarthritis	L- Violet R- Yellow
3.	**Bl54** L&R outside leg hip bone just ↓ tail	Hip joint pain, pelvic limb lameness, muscle atrophy, sciatica	L-Green R-Red
4.	**Bl40** L&R on outside & backside of hindleg where it meets body.	LBP, Hips, Stifles, incontinence, AI disorders, spondylosis, paralysis	L-Green R-Red
5.	**Sp10** L&R inside hindleg opposite hip where leg meets body	Blood deficiency, fever	L-Blue R-Orange
6.	**Sp9** L&R inside hindleg ↓ hip joint in depression above calf muscle.	Incontinence, stifle pain, edema	L-Blue R-Orange
7.	**St41** L&R outside hindleg inside hock joint	Seizures, depression, constipation, hock facial pain, Hip & leg issues	L-Blue R-Orange

General Indications: For hip pain and degeneration

Directions: Shine colored light 15-20 seconds per point. Also perform the Diamond Joint directly over the hip. The most tender of the 4 points is in Green for 20 seconds & the other 3 points are in Red. (See diagram). This treatment is worth diamonds! You can do this on people as well, any joint. TCM (Traditional Chinese Medicine) says you treat one joint, you treat them all.

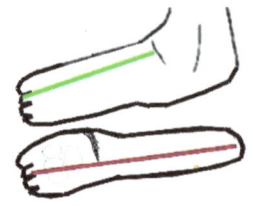

💧 Eases tension in joints, spine. Red on underside of back paw. Green on top of back paw. Stroke lines back & forth 30 seconds each on both back paws.

Insomnia (HtSI)

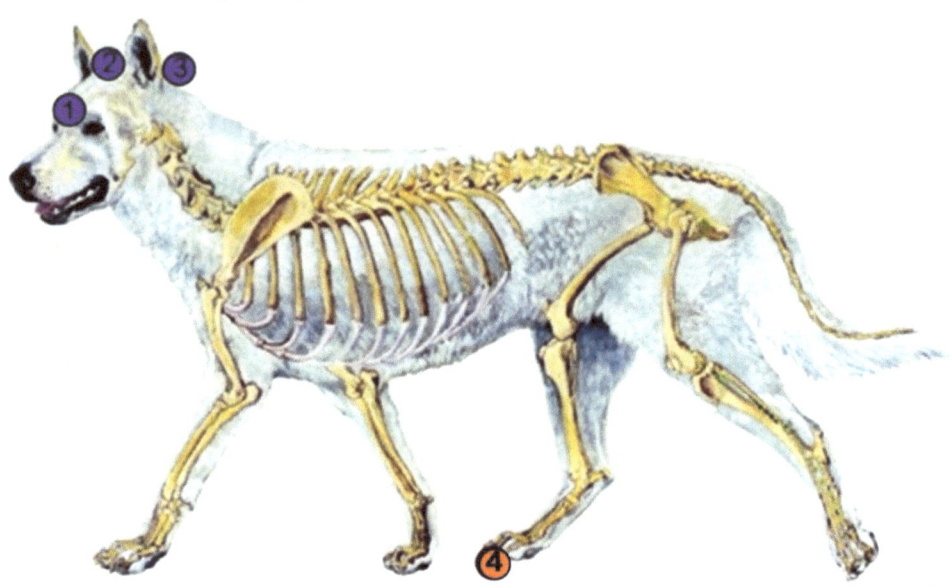

Signs: fatigue during the day, excessive wakefulness during the night. *Nocturnal animals would be just the opposite.

	Location	Indications	Color
1.	Yin Trang – Pineal gland. Between eyebrows	Sleep and Melatonin production, anxiety	Violet
2.	GV20 top head; ↑ from top of ears	Pituitary issues, Diabetes, neck stiffness, insomnia, shock, seizures	Violet
3.	GV16 back crown of head or end of occiput	Epilepsy, stroke, eye vision, hearing DDD	Violet or UV
4.	Sp1 L&R inside hindleg paw 2nd digit	Abdominal pain, distension, anorexia, shock, seizures	L-Blue R-Orange

General Indications: For sleeplessness, fatigue, insufficient melatonin production, anxiety, pituitary issues.

Directions: Shine colored light 15-20 seconds per point.

💧 Lavender is a great essential oil for insomnia. Rub a little behind the ears or on the temples.

Jaw Problems (SpSt)

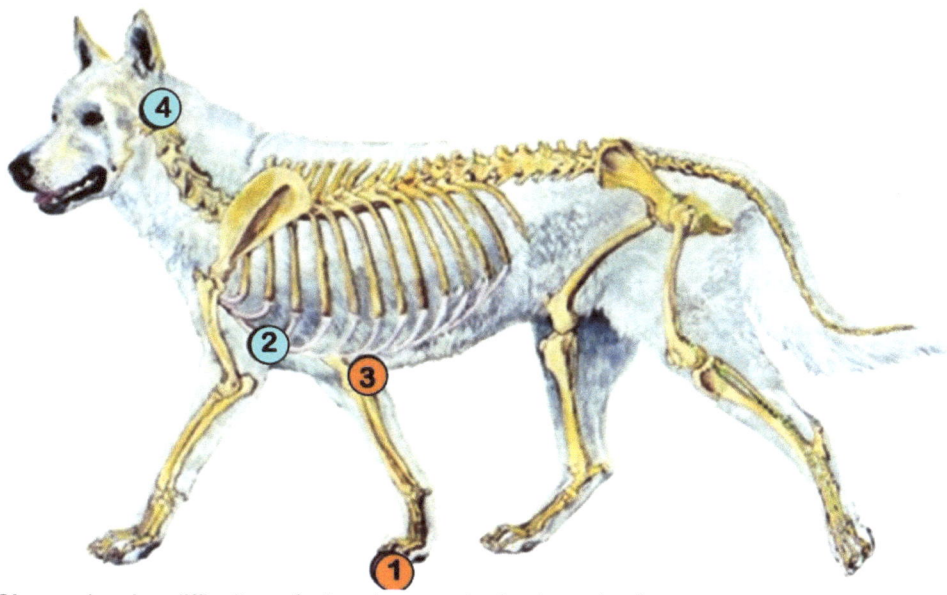

Signs: chewing difficulty, refusing dry crunchy foods or dog bones

	Location	Indications	Color
1.	**LI4** L&R inside forepaw in web between dewclaw & toe 1	Immune mediated skin issues. Sore throat, Cough, Neck, Shoulder pain, Lameness, Fever. Not for PG	L-Blue R-Orange
2.	**Th10** outside frontleg where it meets body	Neck, dental, ear pain, limb paralysis	L-Turquoise R-Orange
3.	**Lu5** L&R front leg at joint where inside front leg meets body	Immune-mediated skin disorders, fever, n/v, diarrhea, shoulder & elbow pain.	L-Blue R-Orange
4.	**TH17** L&R 2FW ↓bottom of ears	Ear disorders, seizures, TMJ & neck pain	L-Turquoise R-Orange

General Indications: For TMJ, inability to chew, toothache, ear pain.

Directions: Shine colored light 15-20 seconds per point.

Liver/Gall Bladder Problems (LvGB)

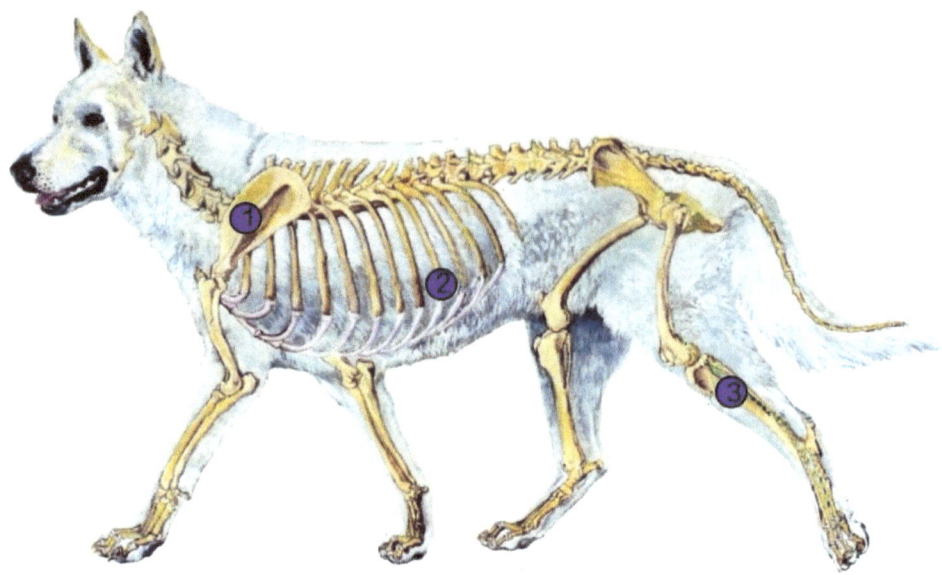

Signs: yellow color on whites of eyes; anorexia, n/v, diarrhea, weight loss, fatigue, ↑urination, excessive thirst, abdominal pain & distention, fever

	Location	Indications	Color
1.	**GB21** L&R sides of scapula, level of C7-T1	Shoulder & back pain. Li/GB disorders, expedites labor, lactation.	L- Violet R- Yellow
2.	**GB24** L&R sides at 9th IC space on ribcage	Expels GB stones, shoulder pain, fatigue	L- Violet R- Yellow
3.	**GB34** L&R outside hindleg 2FW↓hipjoint where meets body	Blood flow, hypertension, n/v, Li/GB disorders, stomach & liver stagnation, pain relief	L- Violet R- Yellow

General Indications: For detoxifying the liver, expelling Gallstones, and any Liver/GB disorders.

Directions: Shine colored light 15-20 seconds per point.

Pain

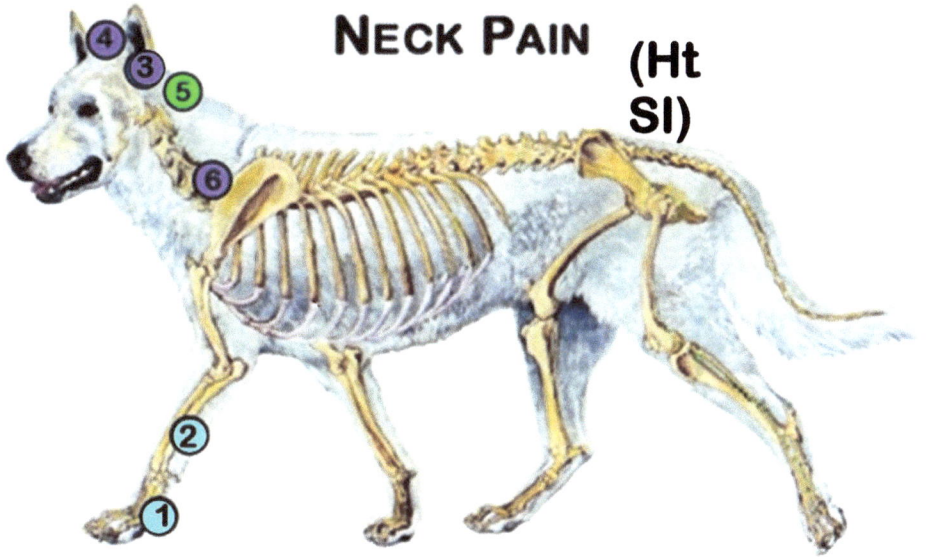

Signs: resists touch, climbing, sitting, getting up/down difficulty, uneven gait, lays down mostly

	Location	Indications	Color
	NECK PAIN		
1.	**SI3** L&R Outside frontleg wrist joint	Fever, conjunctivitis, neck & shoulder pain, epilepsy.	L Turquoise R Pink *
2.	**TH8** L&R outside frontleg 3FW↑ elbow	Foreleg, neck, thoracic, limb, shoulder pain & tension	L-Turquoise R- Orange
3.	**GB20** bottom base of ear	Epilepsy, eye & neck issues	L- Violet R- Yellow
4.	**GV20** top head; ↑ from top of ears	Pituitary issues, Diabetes, neck stiffness, insomnia, shock, seizures	Violet
5.	**Bl10** 3FW each side of spine at C2 or base of head	Eyes, sinuses, Neck & Back Pain, epilepsy, DDD	L-Green R-Red
6.	**GV14** between C7 &T1 on spine	Fever, cough, neck pain, spondylosis, immune system.	Violet

SHOULDER PAIN (HTSI)

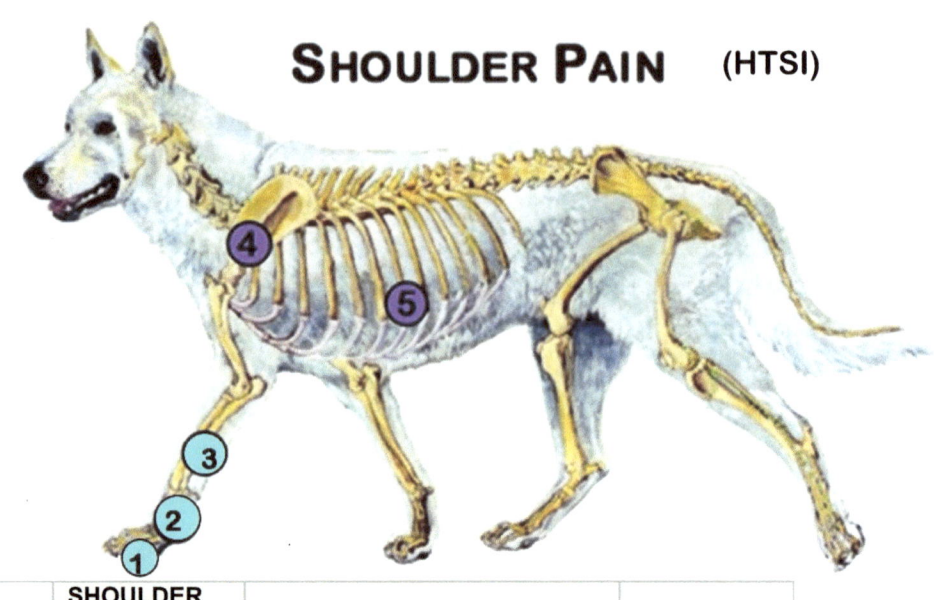

	SHOULDER PAIN		
1.	**TH1** L&R outside front paw at 4th nailbed	Fever, conjunctivitis, deafness, tinnitus, shoulder pain	L-Turquoise R- Orange
2.	**TH4** L&R outside frontleg just ↓elbow	Fatigue, swelling & pain of front paw & shoulder, Diabetes	L-Turquoise R- Orange
3.	**TH8** L&R outside frontleg 3FW↑ elbow	Foreleg, neck, thoracic, limb, shoulder pain & tension	L-Turquoise R- Orange
4.	**GB21** L&R sides of scapula, level of C7-T1	Shoulder & back pain. Li/GB disorders, expedites labor, lactation.	L- Violet R- Yellow
5.	**GB24** L&R sides at 9th IC space on ribcage	Expels GB stones, shoulder pain, fatigue	L- Violet R- Yellow

LOW BACK PAIN (KIBL)

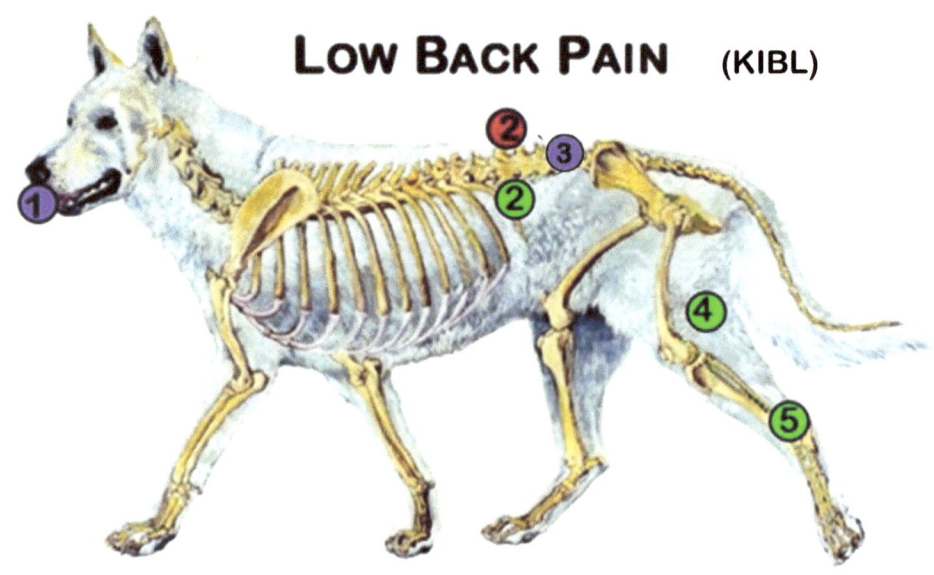

	LOW BACK PAIN (LBP)		
1.	**GV26** mid upper lip	Shock, heatstroke, coma, seizures, spinal pain	Violet
2.	**BI23** 3FW each side of L2	Weakness, seizures, ears, eyes, LBP, kidney, focus, brain	L-Green R-Red
3.	**GV4** on spine at L5	Bone & spine disorders, epilepsy, infertility, diarrhea	Violet or UV
4.	**BI40** L&R on outside & backside of hindleg where it meets body.	LBP, Hips, Stifles, incontinence, AI disorders, spondylosis, paralysis	L-Green R-Red
5.	**BI60** on outside & backside of L&R hindleg ↑hock joint.	LBP, hocks, hypertension, not for PG	L-Green R-Red

LIMB PAIN (LULI)

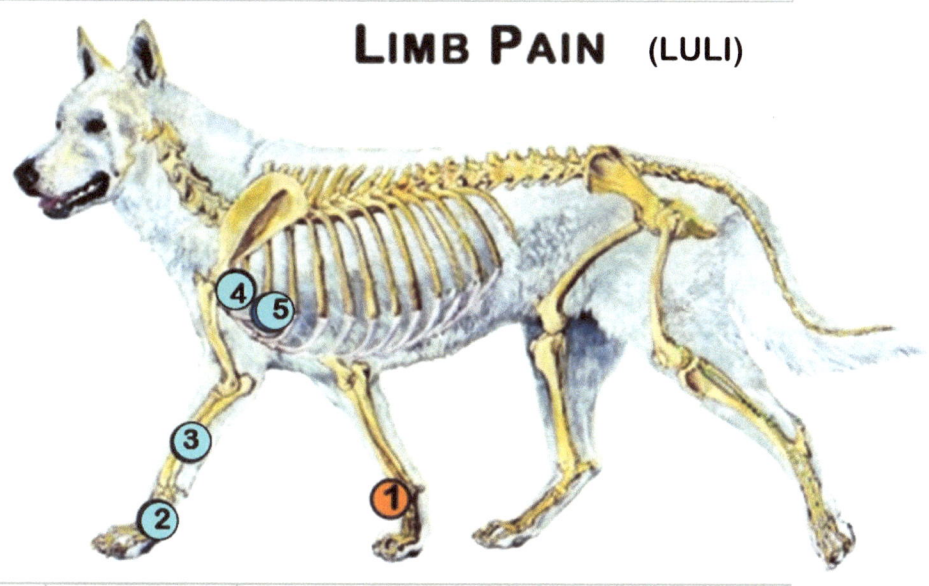

	LIMB PAIN		
1.	**Pc3**- L&R inside frontleg crease of elbow	Heatstroke, fever, palpitations, shoulder & elbow pain, diarrhea	L-Turquoise R- Orange
2.	**TH4** L&R outside frontleg just ↓elbow	Fatigue, swelling & pain of front paw & shoulder, Diabetes	L-Turquoise R- Orange
3.	**TH8** L&R outside frontleg 3FW↑elbow,	Foreleg, neck, thoracic, limb, shoulder pain & tension	L-Turquoise R- Orange
4.	**TH14** L&R base of neck at 1st rib	Shoulder, thoracic, limb pain	L-Turquoise R- Orange
5.	**SI9** L&R at end of 2nd rib on front shoulder joint	Pain, stiffness, paralysis, arthritis of scapula, shoulder, neck & forearm. Inflammation	L Turquoise R Pink *

OTHER HEAD PAIN (HTSI)

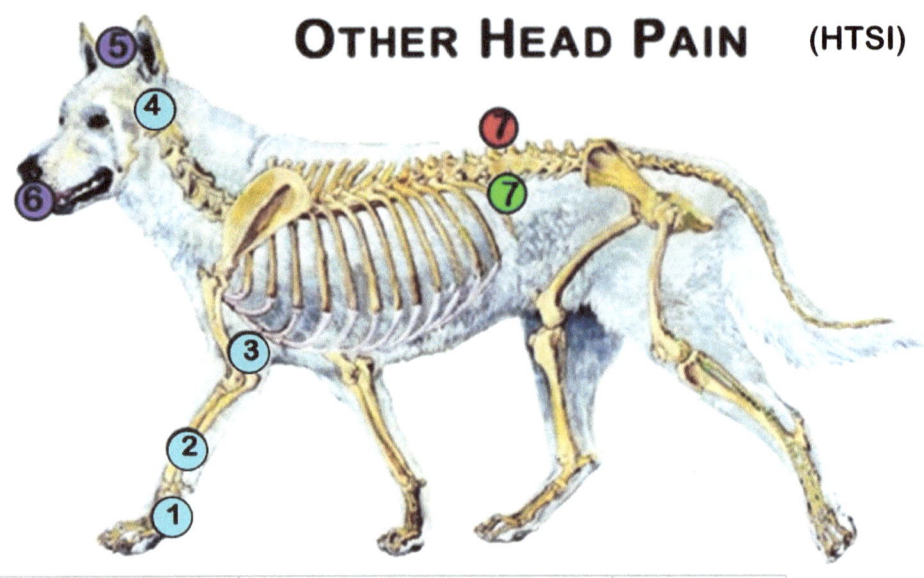

	OTHER HEAD PAIN		
1.	**TH3** L&R outside frontleg 2FW↑paw	Ear, eye issues, fever, shoulder pain	L-Turquoise R- Orange
2.	**TH5** L&R outside frontleg 2FW↑ elbow joint	Otitis, conjunctivitis, fever, shoulder & neck pain, lameness	L-Turquoise R- Orange
3.	**Th10** outside frontleg where it meets body	Neck, dental, ear pain, limb paralysis	L-Turquoise R- Orange
4.	**TH17** L&R 2FW ↓bottom of ears	Ear disorders, seizures, TMJ & neck pain	L-Turquoise R- Orange
5.	**GV20** top head; ↑ from top of ears	Pituitary issues, Diabetes, neck stiffness, insomnia, shock, seizures	Violet
6.	**GV26** mid upper lip	Shock, heatstroke, coma, seizures, spinal pain	Violet
7.	**Bl23** 3FW each side of L2	Weakness, seizures, ears, eyes, LBP, kidney, focus, brain	L-Green R-Red

General Indications: For any pain in body, post-surgical, post-injury, arthritis.

Directions: Choose the acupoints for the affected area—neck, shoulder, limb, dental, TMJ, thoracic & LBP, . Shine colored light 15-20 seconds per point.

- **Essential Oils**—Helichrysum and Roman Chamomile soothe pain

- Eases tension in joints, spine. Red on underside of back paw. Green on top of back paw. Stroke lines back & forth 30 seconds each on both back paws.

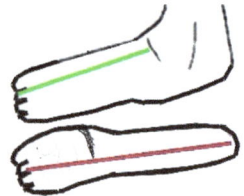

Parasites (SpSt)

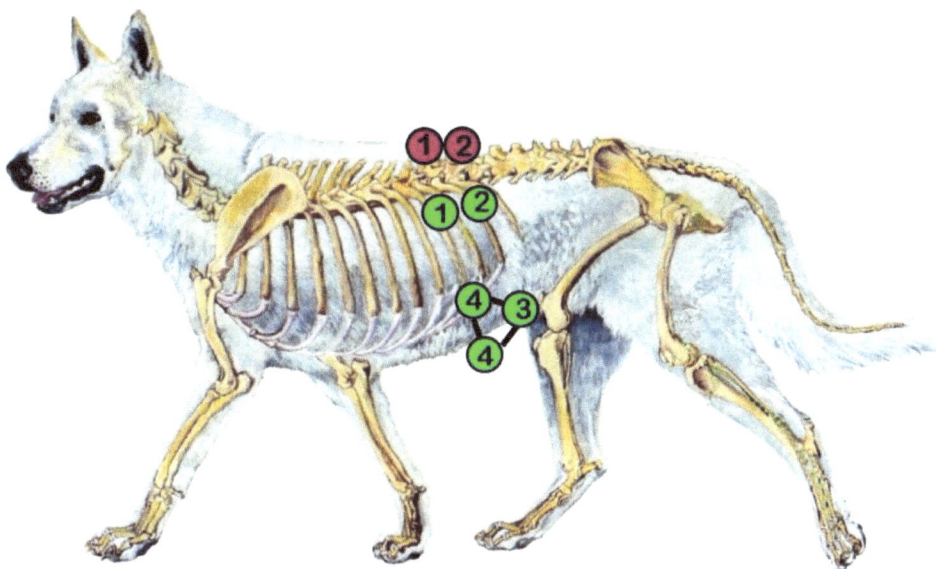

Signs: weight loss, anorexia, weakness, fatigue; dragging bottom on floor; excessive licking of anus

	Location	Indications	Color
1.	**Bl19** 3FW L&R of T11	Fever, eye disorder, sciatica, DDD, Expels Parasites	L-Green R-Red
2.	**Bl20** 3FW L&R of T12	Edema, diarrhea, anemia, GI disorders, abdominal masses	L-Green R-Red
3.	**CV6** 2FW↓ navel	Chronic diarrhea, weakness, constipation, abdominal pain	Green
4.	**St25** 3FW each side of navel	GI disorders, abdominal masses, diarrhea or constipation, n/v	Green

General Indications: For expelling parasites from the body.

Directions: Shine colored light 15-20 seconds per point. Please note that points 4 & 5 are **all** in Green. The color green cools and neutralizes GI infection and discomfort. The 3-point triangle also has a calming effect upon the entire abdominal region.

Neuter/Spay Recovery (LuLI)

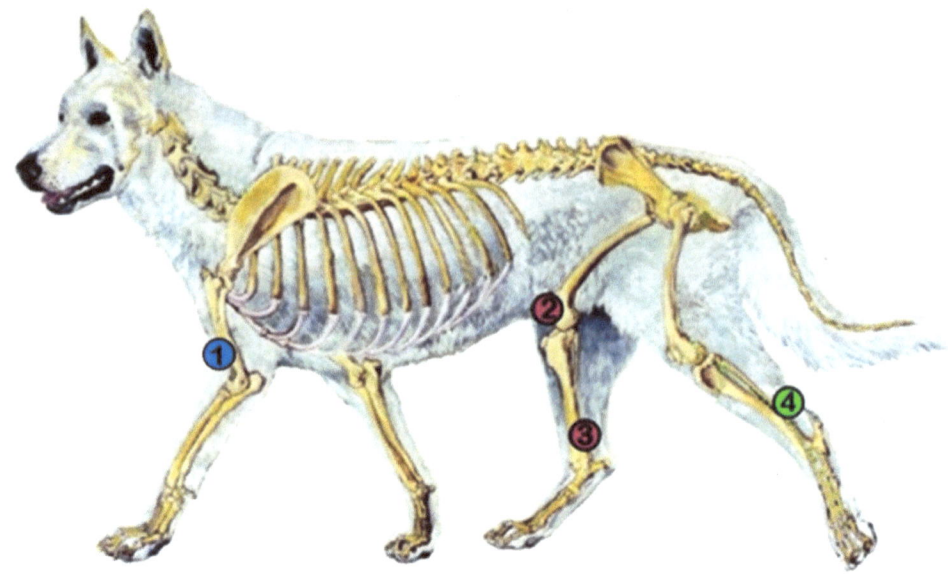

Signs: fatigue and pain after surgery

	Location	Indications	Color
1.	**LI11** L&R front leg at joint where outside front leg meets body	Skin disorders, allergy, fever, endocrine, elbow & foreleg issues	L-Blue R-Orange
2.	**CV4** 4FW↓navel	Weakness, urine retention, diarrhea or infertility	Red or IR
3.	**Ki3** L&R inside hindleg 1FW↑hock joint.	Kidney issues & renal failure, arthritis, hock swelling, LBP, ears, PMS	L-Green R-Red
4.	**Bl60** on outside & backside of L&R hindleg ↑hock joint.	LBP, hocks, hypertension, not for PG	L-Green R-Red

General Indications: For post-surgical procedures to help with recovery

Directions: Shine colored light 15-20 seconds per point.

Respiratory Problems (LuLI)

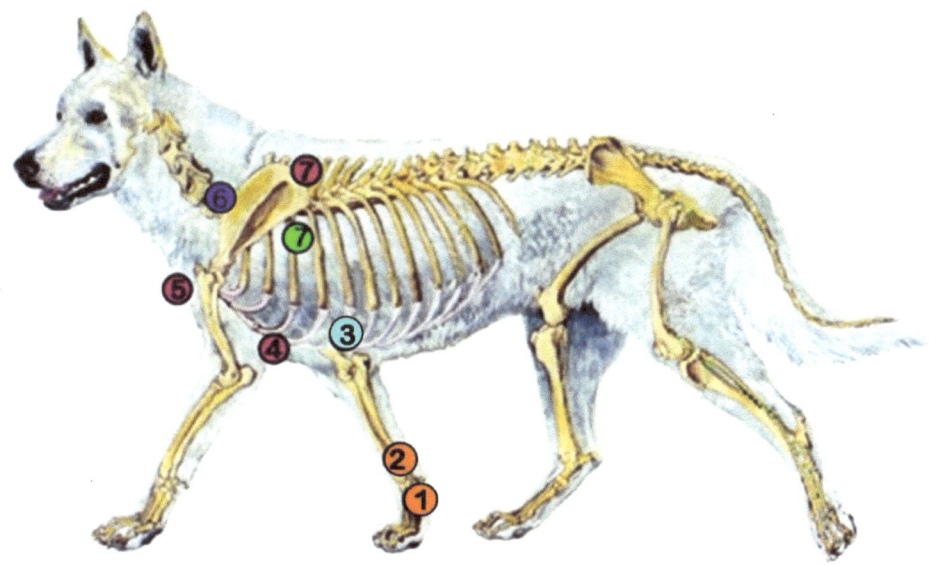

Signs: Sneezes, wheezes, coughs & foams, short of breath, pants, discharge eyes or nose, blue around lips, gums, tongue; fever, no appetite

	Location	Indications	Color
1.	**Lu7** L&R outside front leg just above radial wrist joint	Asthma, cough, neck, toothache	L -Blue R- Orange
2.	**Lu9** L&R inside frontleg 1FW↓ elbow joint	Chest pain, asthma, cough, shoulder & back pain, front leg pain, heatstroke, coma	L -Blue R- Orange
3.	**Pc1** L&R 4FW↓ IC5 space	Expands chest, cough, fatigue, lactation, mastitis	L-Turquoise R- Orange
4.	**CV17** midline outside frontleg where it meets body	Cough, vomiting, lactation	Red
5.	**CV20** on neck midline at 1st IC space	Cough, respiratory issues, difficulty breathing	Red
6.	**GV14** between C7 &T1 on spine	Fever, cough, cervical pain, spondylosis, immune system.	Violet
7.	**Bl13** 3FW L&R of T3	Sadness, Respiratory issues, neck or back stiffness	L-Green R-Red

General Indications: For asthma, bronchitis, sinusitis and other Lung/Large Intestine issues..

Directions: Shine colored light 15-20 seconds per point.

Reproduction Problems (LuLI)

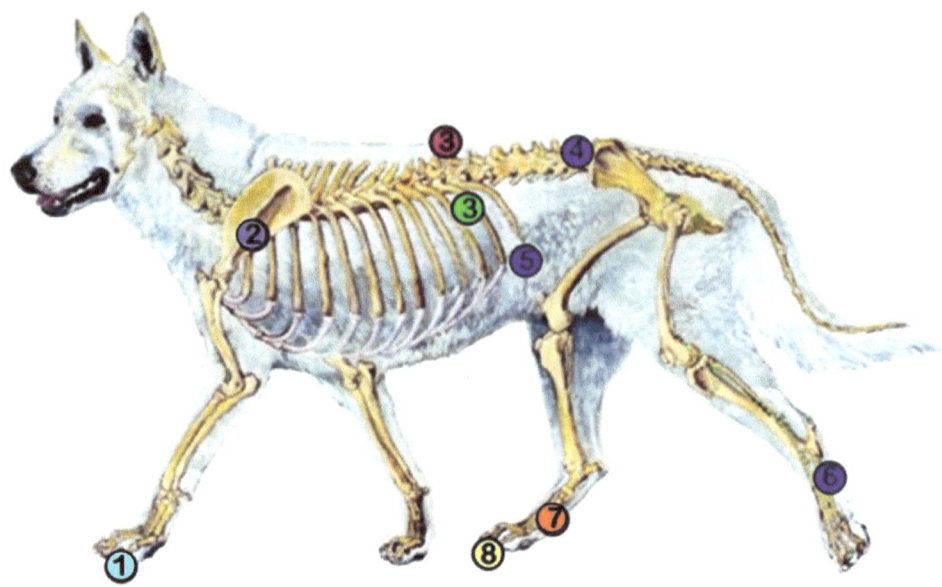

Signs: Irregular period, difficult labor, lactation issues

	Location	Indications	Color
1.	SI1 L&R outside 5th toe front paws	Fever, coma, shoulder pain, lactations	L Turquoise R Pink *
2.	GB21 L&R sides of scapula, level of C7-T1	Shoulder & back pain. Li/GB disorders, expedites labor, lactation.	L- Violet R- Yellow
3.	Bl20 3FW L&R of T12	Edema, diarrhea, anemia, GI disorders, abdominal masses	L-Green R-Red
4.	GV4 on spine at L5	Bone & spine disorders, epilepsy, infertility, diarrhea	Violet or UV
5.	Lv13 L&R at lowest point 12th rib on sides	Fatigue, Abdominal pain & Distention, Swelling of legs	L- Violet R- Yellow
6.	GB41 4FW↓hock joint	Eye pain, irregular cycles, hip pain, lactation	L- Violet R- Yellow
7.	Sp4 L&R inside hindleg 2FW↑ankle	Indigestion, abdominal pain, diarrhea, irregular cycles	L -Blue R- Orange
8.	Lv2 L&R inside hindleg on 2nd toe of paw	Eye, PMS, incontinence or retention, epilepsy	L- Violet R- Yellow

General Indications: For balancing chi energy in Reproduction difficulties.

Directions: Shine colored light 15-20 seconds per point.

Sadness or Grief (LuLI)

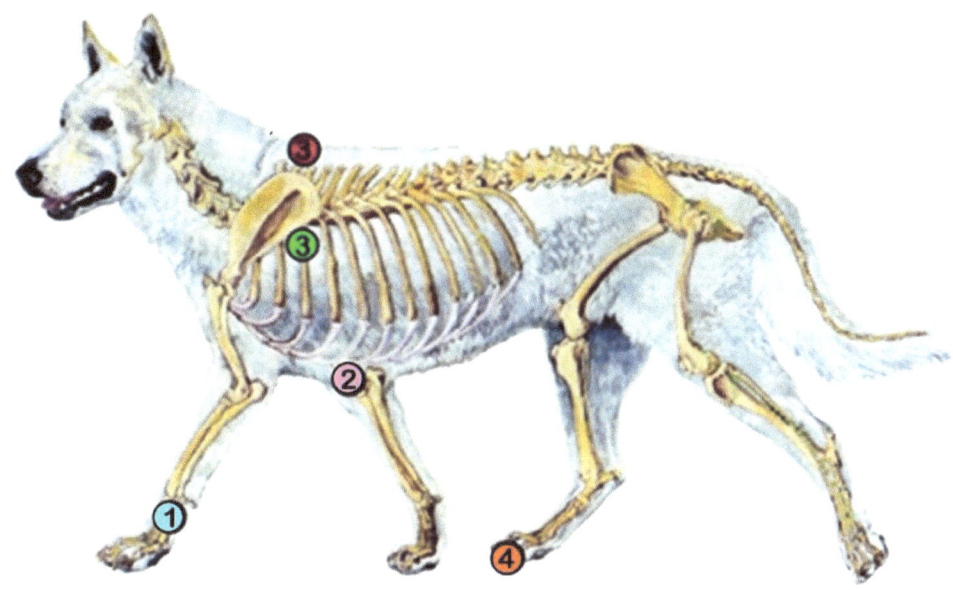

Signs: sad, dull eyes, not eating

	Location	Indications	Color
1.	**TH3** L&R outside frontleg 2FW↑paw	Ear, eye issues, fever, shoulder pain	L-Turquoise R- Orange
2.	**Ht1** L&R inside frontleg center of armpit	Chest & shoulder pain, hysteria, impulsiveness, & depression	L Turquoise R Pink *
3.	**Bl13** 3FW L&R of T3	Sadness, Respiratory issues, neck or back stiffness	L-Green R-Red
4.	**Sp1** L&R inside hindleg paw 2nd digit	Abdominal pain, distension, anorexia, shock, seizures	L-Blue R-Orange

General Indications: For sadness and depression and other Lung/Large Intestinal issues.

Directions: Shine colored light 15-20 seconds per point.

💧 **Essential oils**—Roman Chamomile, Valerian Root, & Lavender help with grief.

Sedation (KiBl)

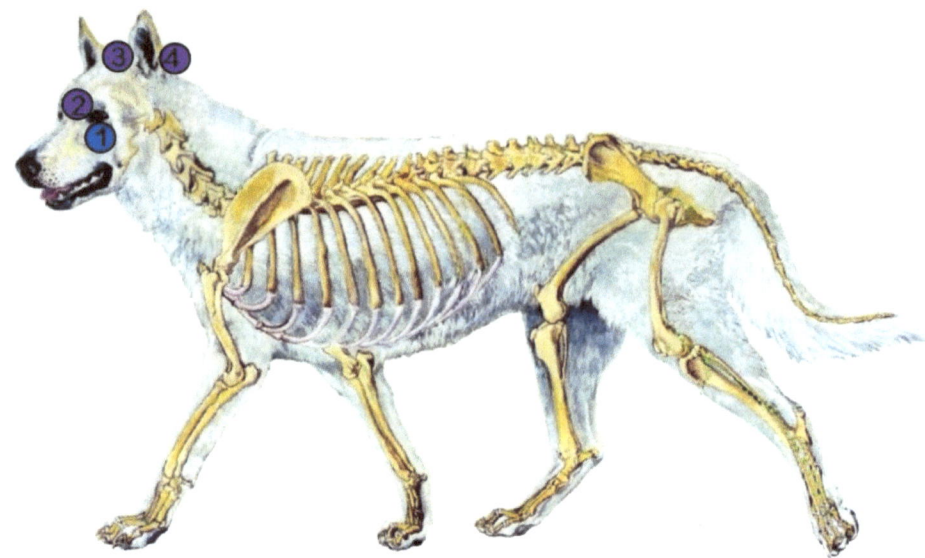

Signs: Anxiousness, hesitation or resistance

	Location	Indications	Color
1.	**St1** L&R under pupil of eye	Conjunctivitis, uveitis, discharge, swelling excessive tearing	L -Blue R- Orange
2.	**Yin Trang** – Pineal gland. Between eyebrows	Sleep and Melatonin production, anxiety	Violet
3.	**GV20** top head; ↑ from top of ears	Pituitary issues, Diabetes, neck stiffness, insomnia, shock, seizures	Violet
4.	**GV19** at the crown of the head before occiput tapers down	Clears trauma, insomnia, seizures, pituitary issues, neck pain, shock	Violet

General Indications: For relaxation before or after surgery, travel, etc.

Directions: Shine colored light 15-20 seconds per point.

Throat/Thyroid Conditions (LuLI)

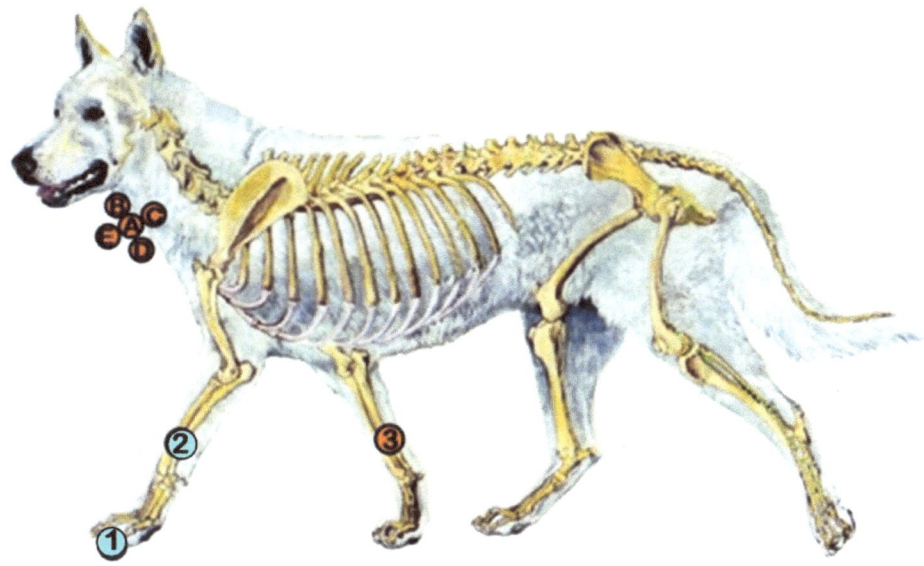

Signs: inability to swallow foods, fatigue, weight change, dull coat, hair loss

	Location	Indications	Color
1.	**TH1** L&R outside front paw at 4th nailbed	Fever, conjunctivitis, deafness, tinnitus, shoulder pain	L-Turquoise R- Orange
2.	**TH5** L&R outside frontleg 2FW↑ elbow joint	Otitis, conjunctivitis, fever, shoulder & neck pain, lameness	L-Turquoise R- Orange
3.	**Pc5** L&R inside frontleg 4FW↑ elbow joint	Seizures, severe agitation, n/v, palpitations	L-Turquoise R- Orange
4.	Thyroid Cross. Midpoint mid thyroid. Then points BCDE	Hypothyroidism	Orange

General Indications: For inflammation or infection of throat, thyroid issues, neck & shoulder pain

Directions: Shine colored light 15-20 seconds per point. The Thyroid Cross is a great way to regulate the thyroid (the Adam's apple in the middle of the throat) when it is under/over active. Use orange for hypothyroidism (underactive) and turquoise for hyperthyroidism (overactive).

Toothaches (LuLI)

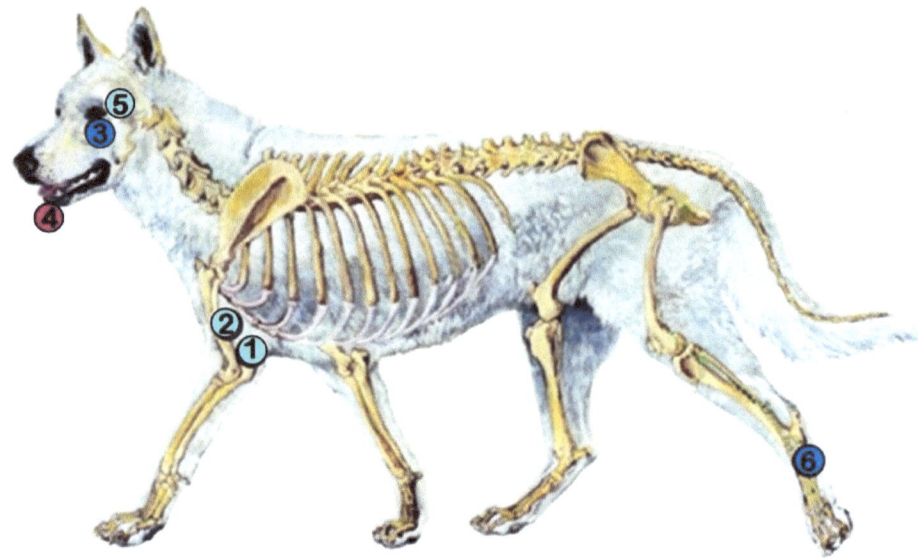

Signs: difficulty to chew dog biscuits or dry dogfood without pain, more than usual drooling, gums inflamed, tooth abscess; dirty, stained, worn or broken teeth; gums Inflamed.

	Location	Indications	Color
1.	SI8 Outside frontleg at joint where leg meets body	Elbow pain, seizures, neck, shoulder & teeth pain.	L Turquoise R Pink *
2.	Th10 outside frontleg where it meets body	Neck, dental, ear pain, limb paralysis	L-Turquoise R- Orange
3.	St1 L&R under pupil of eye	Conjunctivitis, uveitis, discharge, swelling excessive tearing	L -Blue R- Orange
4.	CV24 center lower lip	Behavioral disorders, mania, seizures, gingivitis, gum or tooth pain	Red or IR
5.	TH23 L&R end of eyebrow in hole	Epilepsy, eye disorders, dental issues, facial paralysis	L-Turquoise R- Orange
6.	St42 L&R outside hindleg2FW↓hock	Toothaches, gingivitis, n/v	L -Blue R- Orange

General Indications: For dental disease and pain Check individual teeth using APPENDIX 3

Directions: Shine colored light 15-20 seconds per point. When a particular tooth is troublesome and painful, look to the related meridian for an allergy or imbalance, since some of the major meridians pass through the gum and dental areas. Use Appendix 3:the Dental Connection APPENDIX 3: Dental Connection

Trauma, Emotional and Physical (HtSI)

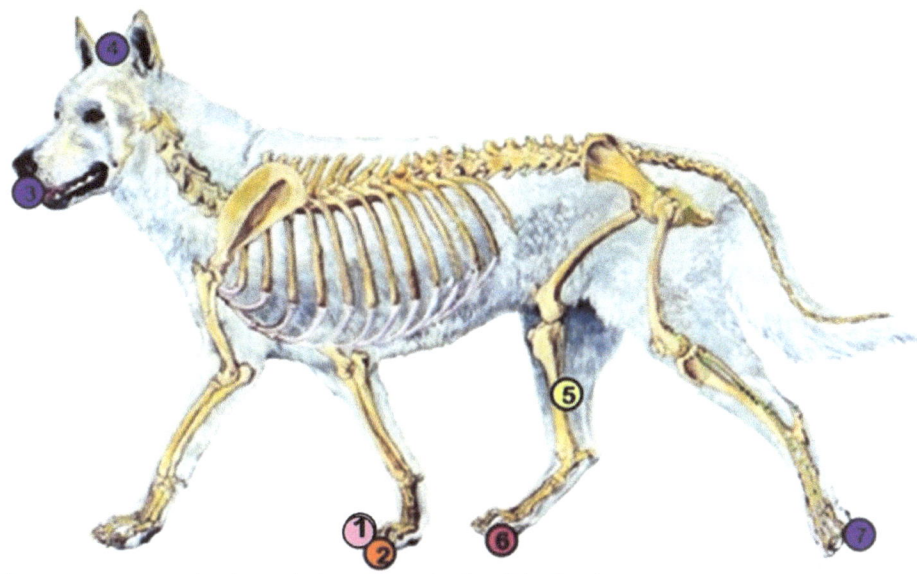

Signs: nonresponsive to verbal commands, fearful, shock, anger,

	Location	Indications	Color
1.	**Ht9** L&R inside front leg at 5th toe of paw	Revives LOC, regulates heart, fever, shoulder & neck issues	L Turquoise R Pink *
2.	**Pc9** L&R inside frontleg at nailbed, 3rd digit	Confusion, shock, LOC, heatstroke, fever	L-Turquoise R- Orange
3.	**GV26** mid upper lip	Shock, heatstroke, coma, seizures, spinal pain	Violet
4.	**GV20** top head; ↑ from top of ears	Pituitary issues, Diabetes, neck stiffness, insomnia, shock, seizures	Violet
5.	**Lv5** L&R inside hindleg, midway hock to body	LOC, LBP, urinary incontinence, impotence, PMS, sterility	L- Violet R- Yellow
6.	**Ki1** L&R inside hindleg on 1st toe of paw	Incontinence, infertility, heatstroke, fever	L-Green R-Red
7.	**GB44** L&R outside paw of hindleg at 4th nailbed	Fever, hypertension, shock, eye issues	L- Violet R- Yellow

General Indications: For negative emotions and resulting physical issues

Directions: Shine colored light 15-20 seconds per point.

♪ This Trauma Treatment has been very effective on my 2 year old granddaughter. She came home from her dad's one day and hid under a table. The next couple of days she wouldn't take a nap on her bed, and she had to have me beside her until she fell asleep. Once we used this treatment, she was back to her usual self, because the emotional trauma was released. The next day she resumed her naps on her own. As she talked more and more, she told us that she was afraid of her Pap-pa. It is very unfortunate that animals and young children experience such emotional trauma, but it is also reassuring that we have a way of releasing it before it scars their physical health.

○ Pink underside of back paw. Sky Blue or Turquoise on top part of back paw.

SECTION III: BALANCING THE MERIDIANS

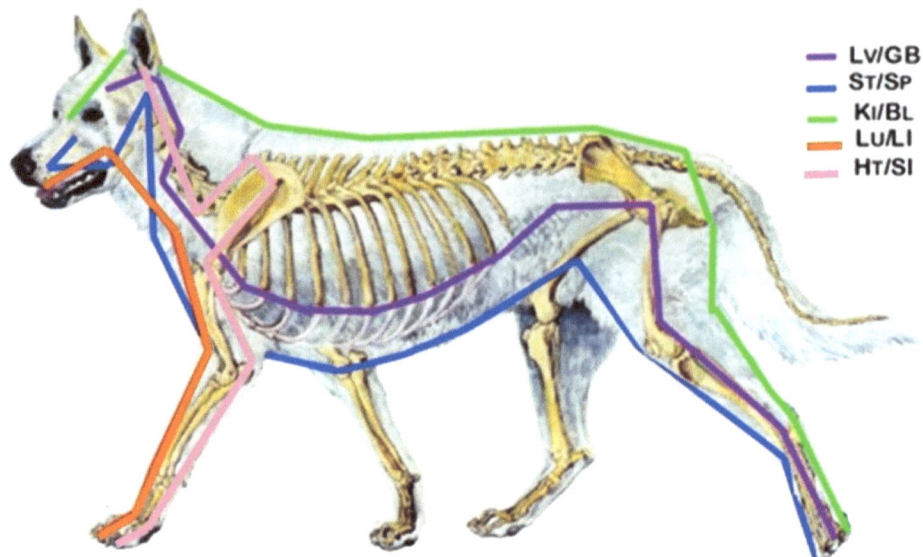

Meridians are energy pathways that link the outside physical body to the inside spirit body. The meridians are closely linked to the nervous system and the nerve pathways that feed every organ and part of the body. Balancing the meridians, balances the whole body-soul-spirit.[i]

How do we know when a meridian is out of balance? Simple…Go back to the *Five Paired Meridian Pathways* chart in the *Introduction* and find the physical issues that you have been dealing with. Which meridian category do those fall into? Balance that meridian pair. Also, on the assessment chart find out what meridians are imbalanced from what signs are observed and balance those meridian pairs.

1. **Meridian Alignment**: An easy way to balance all the meridians is using the meridian face points. The points can also be transposed onto the abdomen, if preferred.

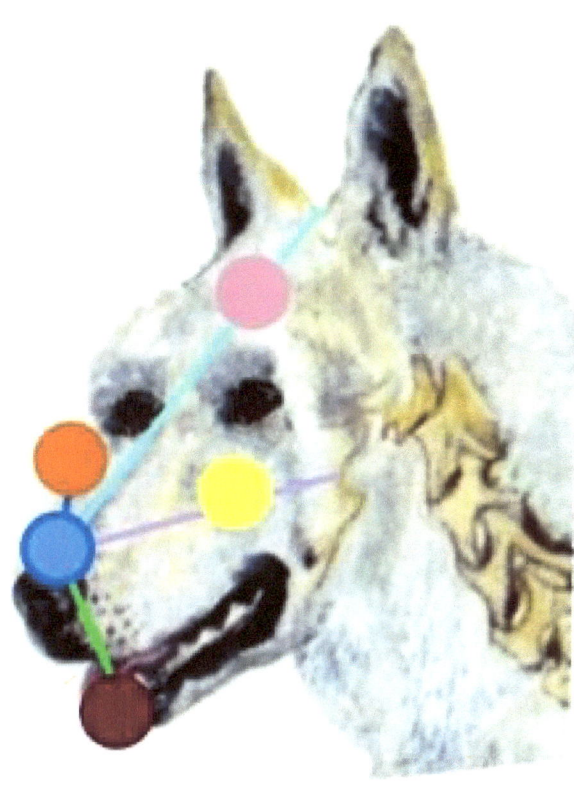

General Indications: This treatment resets all of the meridians. If you are at a loss of where to start due too many symptoms from multiple meridians, use this treatment.

Directions:
1) Treat the Heart point in **Pink** spiraling in and out 20 seconds.
2) Stroke the Heart line in **Turquoise** back and forth 10x from hairline to the spleen.
3) Treat the Liver point in **Yellow** spiraling in and out 20 seconds.
4) Stroke the Liver line in **Violet** back and forth 10x from ear to the spleen.
5) Treat the Kidney point in **Red** spiraling in and out 20 seconds.
6) Stroke the Kidney line in **Green** back and forth 10x from chin to the spleen.
7) Treat the Lung point in **Orange** spiraling in and out 20 seconds.
8) Stroke the Lung line in **Blue** back and forth 10x from ear to the spleen.
9) Treat the Spleen point in **Blue** spiraling in and out 20 seconds

2. **Meridian Tracing**: The energy of the Meridian pairs runs in opposition or Yin and Yang. Normally, the opposing forces keep the meridian pairs balanced, but occasionally the acupoints along one of the meridian pathways become physically or emotionally blocked causing a drop in energy in that pathway, while the opposing compensates with too much. An example of this is when the Liver meridian becomes blocked by anger causing migraines. There is a drop in energy in the Liver meridian which needs to be stimulated using the warm color **Yellow**. The Gall Bladder meridian tries to compensate with too much energy and needs to be sedated using the cool color **Violet**. Start at the **Green** dot and end at the **Red**.

LIVER/GALL BLADDER MERIDIAN

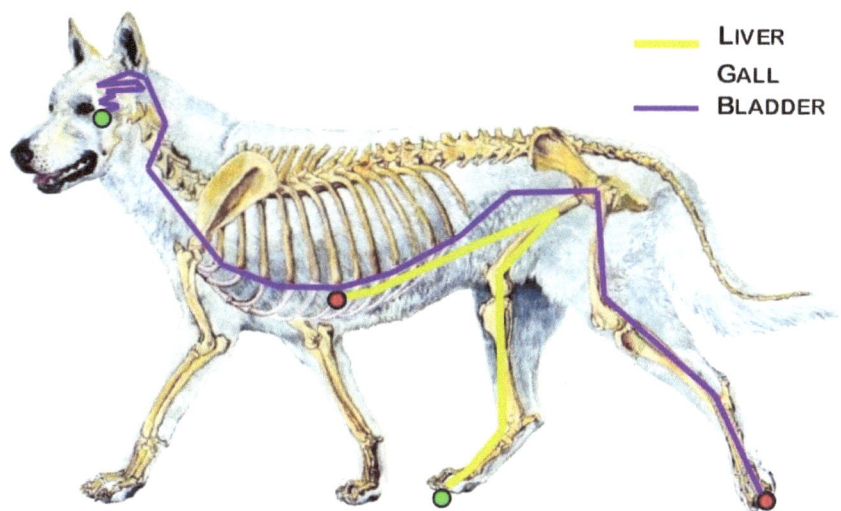

Anger is a powerful emotion that may produce migraine HAs, eye problems, myopathy or tendinitis.

Meridian	Underactive Warm Color	Overactive Cool Color
Liver	Yellow	Violet
Gall Bladder	Yellow	Violet

STOMACH/SPLEEN MERIDIAN

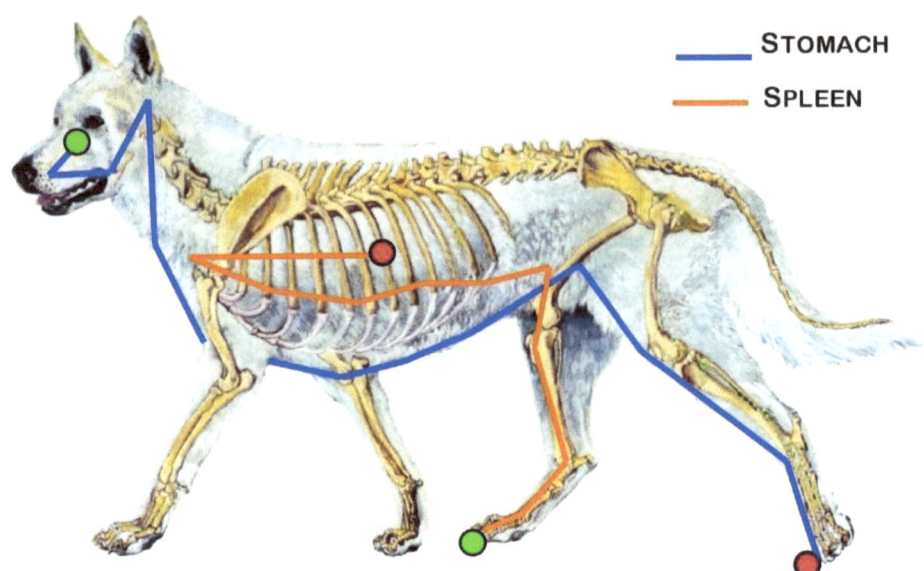

— STOMACH
— SPLEEN

Ever heard of the "Worry-Wart" that ends up with stomach ulcers?

Meridian	Underactive Warm Color	Overactive Cool Color
Stomach	Orange	Blue
Spleen	Orange	Blue

KIDNEY/BLADDER MERIDIAN

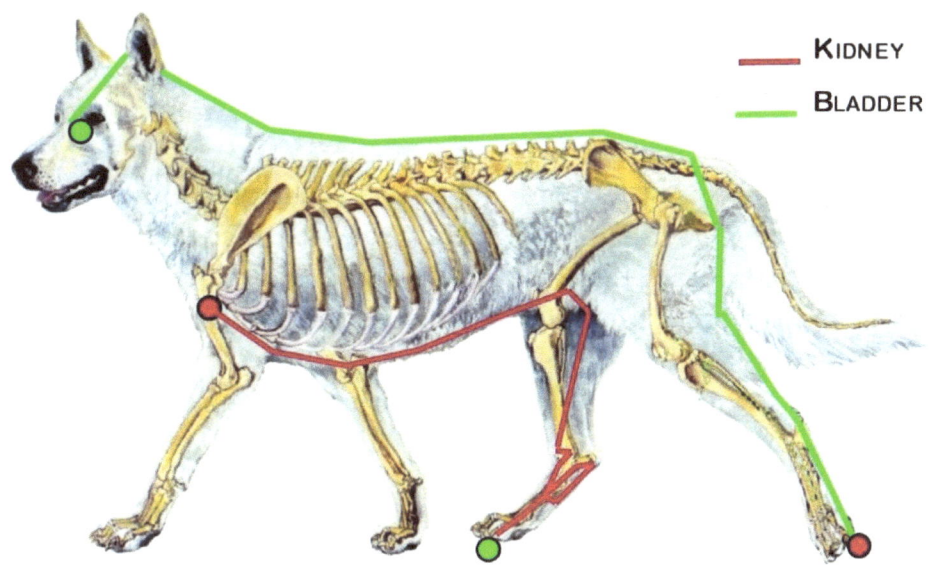

— KIDNEY
— BLADDER

Fear and anxiety are common in young children and can even be transferred from the parents to the unborn child while in the womb. Worry is the acute form of fear and can be released fairly easily. But, once worry develops into anxiety or anxious moments and eventually becomes chronic fear which is much more difficult to release than its more acute forms. Physically, chronic fear causes degeneration of the muscles and joints of the body.

Meridian	Underactive Warm Color	Overactive Cool Color
Kidney	Red	Green
Bladder	Red	Green

An additional step, stroking 5 times on the Kidney/Bladder lines on both feet can clear unwanted prenatal emotion. Everyone should do this *Antepartum treatment* at least once in their course of color therapy.

| 1. Kidney Line | 5x | 3rd toe to heel on bottom of L&R foot | Orange |
| 2. Bladder Line | 5x | 5th toe bunion to heel on side of L&R foot | Yellow |

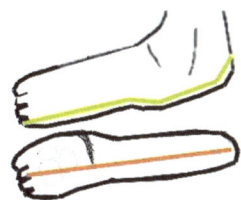

LUNG/LARGE INTESTINE MERIDIAN

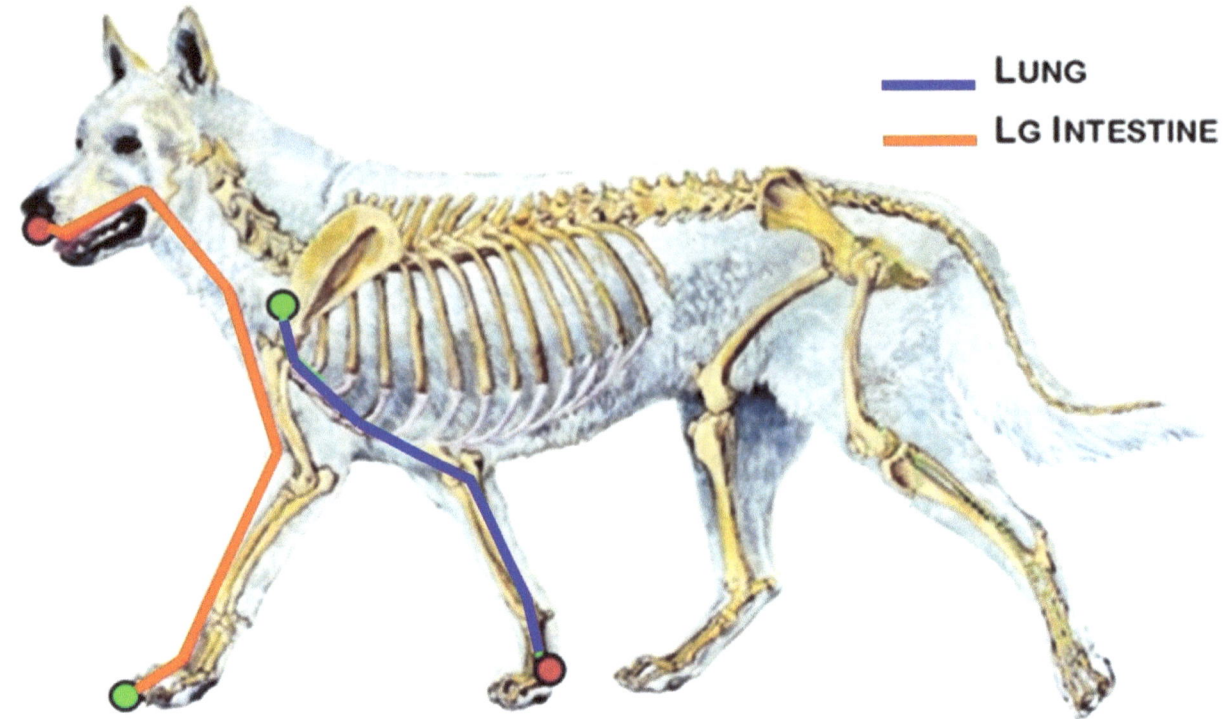

Grief or sorrow will settle in the lungs. Chronic grief becomes depression.

Meridian	Underactive Warm Color	Overactive Cool Color
Lung	Orange	Blue
Large Intestine	Orange	Blue

HEART/SMALL INTESTINE MERIDIAN

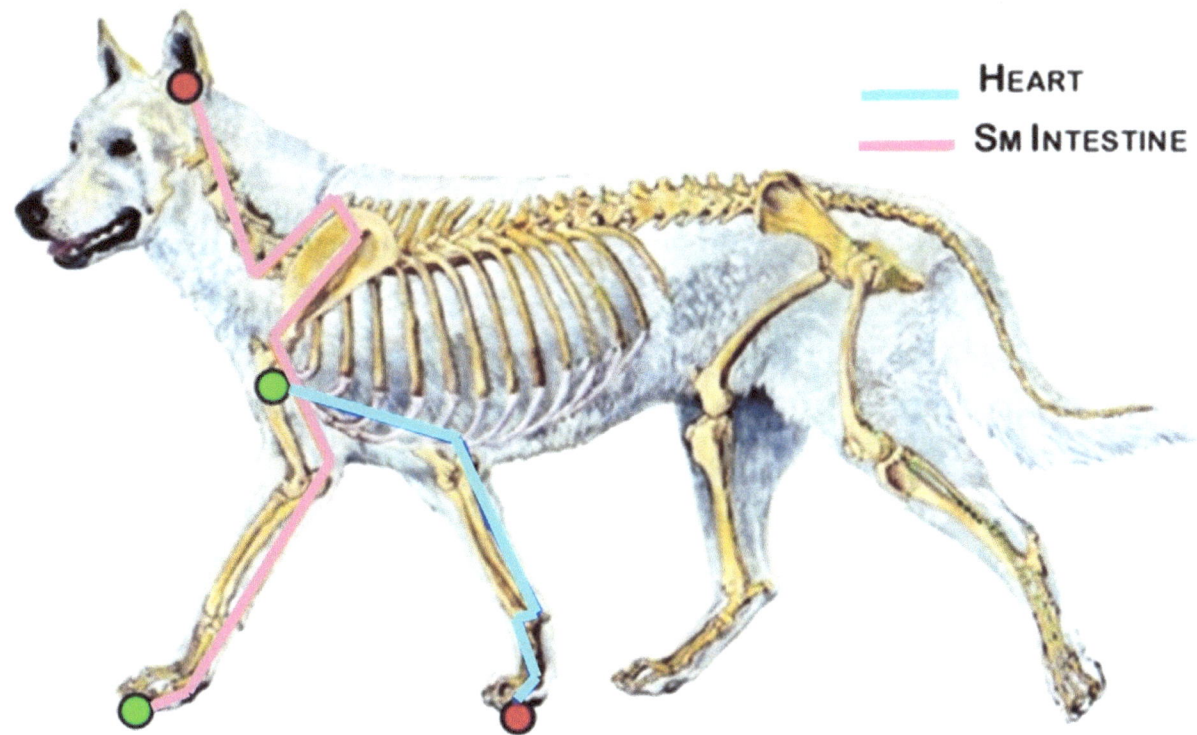

The Heart should be full of Unconditional Love. This meridian should never be out of balance. If it is, then the others are as well, since the other meridians protect the Ht/SI at all costs.

Meridian	Underactive Warm Color	Overactive Cool Color
Heart	Rose	Turquoise
Small Intestine	Rose	Turquoise

CONCLUSION

Taking care of your pet's health doesn't have to be difficult, and certainly we don't have to turn over all of that responsibility to Veterinarians. AcuColors' simple color-by-number treatments are designed to release negative energy and to heal the body-soul-spirit so that it can function-feel-communicate as one whole entity. The main benefit of using AcuColors is that the body either utilizes the color to heal or it doesn't. There are no side effects nor any buildup of toxic substances to damage body tissue, or cause emotional/psychological dependence. What better way is there to heal the body than to use colored light, since animals are also beings of light energy!

The one difference I see in working with animals and small children is that they accept any such help without reservation because they love and trust unconditionally. This is why the treatments work, even instantaneously, for them. As older adults if we have the same faith and trust as we work with Acucolors, we will see the desired results. But realize, that as we age we also store more negative emotions that develop into physical conditions. So essentially, we have to peel back layer upon layer of this negativity in order to be free of the physical diseases; and that takes time. It's the same with rescue animals that have been abused. It takes time to peel back the layers of negativity to heel them emotionally and physically.

In no way do I have all the answers to healing with color or with any of the alternative therapies for that matter. I have simply chosen information for my book from my past experience in hopes that it might help others. Helping others has been my sole purpose in releasing this eBook; and I would hope to publish future sequels as I perfect my treatments and techniques. So, I do solicit feedback since this is how I perfect my information base. Please send feedback to: karen@acucolors.com or go directly to my website: www.acucolors.com and fill in the contact form. Thank you for your suggestions.

APPENDIX 1: FINDING THE RIGHT COLOR TOOLS

Just about any flashlight and color gels will work in applying colored light to the meridian points of the body.

These are just a few ideas so that you can get started.

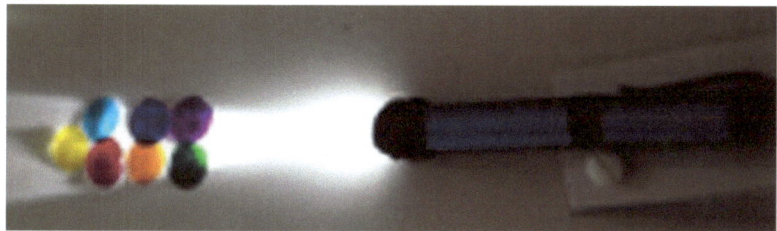

This is an inexpensive bright Rayovac 1AAA penlight with the 7 basic 5/8 " color gels cut to fit into a clear hairspray overcap and then sized with elastic bands to fit tightly over the end of the penlight. The advantage of this penlight is that the switch at the top stays on so you don't have to hold the button down.

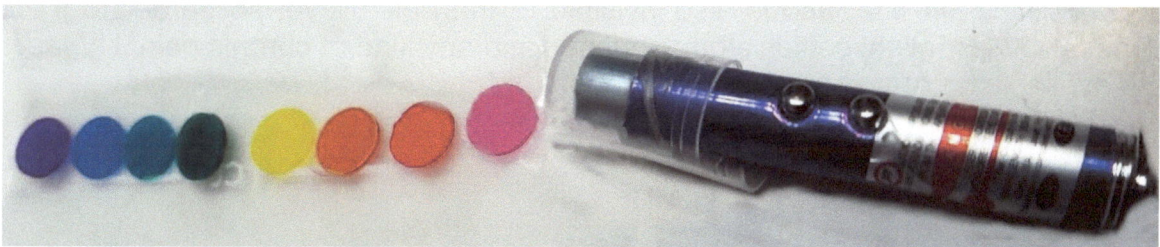

A keychain penlight that fits into a mini overcap is even handier on-the-go. These little penlights with an additional red laser button are available at King Dollar. I keep one of these in my purse because they are so small. The mini overcap comes from Aromaready's glass tube sprayer and holds 3/8" color disks.

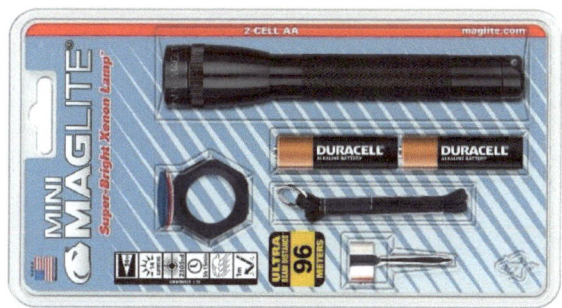
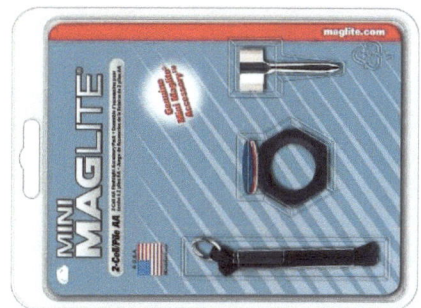

The Mini Maglite combo set $20, or just the accessory kit $10 are available on Amazon. 3 plastic color disks--blue, red, & clear--come with the outer ring that slips over the end of the flashlight. Such durability for less. Simply color the clear disk with a yellow sharpie. Then, cut out the 4 missing spectral colors (Orange, Turquoise, Green and Violet) from gel filter paper, and you have a complete light set. I have yet to work out a deal with Maglite to produce the 4 remaining plastic disks.

https://www.amazon.com/gp/product/B0000AS1G5/ref=ox_sc_sfl_title_1?ie=UTF8&psc=1&smid=ATVPDKIKX0DER

https://www.amazon.com/Maglite-Mini-Flashlight-Accessory-Pack/dp/B00002ND52/ref=pd_sim_469_4?ie=UTF8&dpID=419obIYoj4L&dpSrc=sims&preST=_AC_UL160_SR160%2C160_&refRID=DNT7S4J41PEKBR743F3C

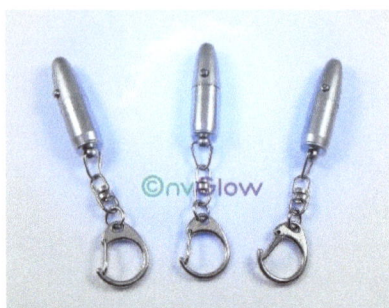

Laser pointer lights are more penetrating than the color gels. Red laser is ideal for moving acute pain and inflammation. These red laser pointers are available at the dollar store. Use it directly on any painful areas for 20-30 seconds. The most penetrating is Infrared (IR) but it is difficult to find, and is also invisible to the naked eye, so harder to track effectiveness. UV laser light settles stomachaches and any kind of chronic pain. UV laser lights are available on Amazon.

https://www.amazon.com/gp/product/B01N9CWKKA/ref=ox_sc_act_title_4?ie=UTF8&psc=1&smid=A23VF2NU5CLMM1

Where can we get Gel Filter paper? Amazon of course! Or any photographic store. They are used to correct lighting during photo shoots. These are sets of colors I have used.

http://www.amazon.com/American-Cgs9A-Precut-Gel-Pack/dp/B0006Z7M46/ref=pd_bxgy_267_img_3?ie=UTF8&refRID=14CVAZ6PE804KPV4CBXR

Or:

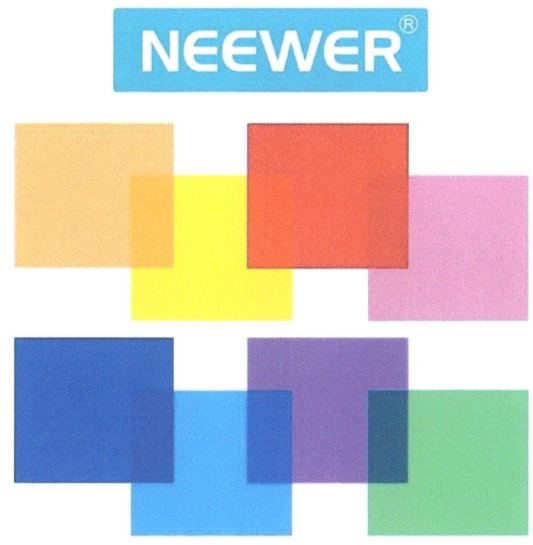

I found this set of plastic gel sheets that has pink included. Some of the colors don't have sufficient dye in them to stop the white light from shining through, but I found that these colors will mix easily, and they are easily corrected. Here is a chart of what I've done to correct these color gels. Punch out and glue together the following disks:

Color	Correction
Red	Ok, but not great. Using a Red laser light is preferred since it penetrates deeper into the cells.
Orange	1 Yellow + 1 Red + 1 of the deficient Orange
Yellow	Ok, but double it for strength
Green	2 of the deficient Green + 1 Light Blue + 1 Yellow
Turquoise	1 Light Blue + 1 Greeng
Indigo	Ok by itself
Violet	3 Violet
Pink	2 Pink makes it stronger
Crimson	1 Red + 3 Violet + 1 Pink (this color has not been defined yet in AcuColors, but may be used at a future date.). It is a great color for pulling out negative emotions.

https://www.amazon.com/gp/product/B01CCIKB5Q/ref=oh_aui_search_detailpage?ie=UTF8&psc=1

Circle Punches... Not all paper punches will cut thru Gel Filters, so start with these EK Tools.

http://www.amazon.com/gp/product/B00C90WM14?psc=1&redirect=true&ref_=ox_sc_act_title_1&smid=ATVPDKIKX0DER

There are also a few professional light tools already out there:

- PERLUX 117 $650
  https://colorpuncture.org/products/light-tools/perlux-p117-light-pen/

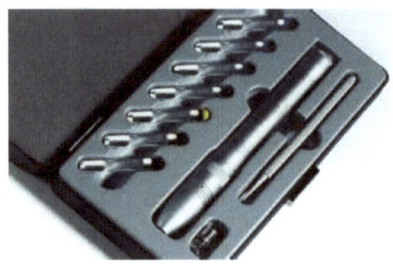

- CHROMOTHERAPY TORCH $200
  http://www.natures-energies.com/natural-therapies/colour-light-therapy-chromotherapy-resources-and-equipment

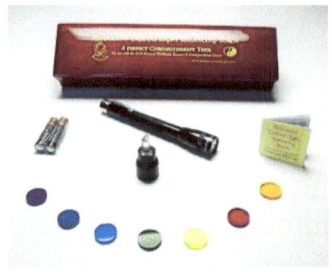

- MOLIMED $400
  http://www.molimed.ch/contents/en-us/d65_molimedpen.html

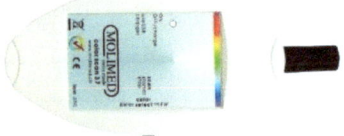

- STREAMLIGHT Penlights $15-25
  http://www.amazon.com/Streamlight-65075-Stylus-Penlight-Green/dp/B0052TJCMQ/ref=sr_1_14?ie=UTF8&qid=1441937017&sr=8-14&keywords=streamlight+pen+light

So, you can see, there are some good color tools available out there depending upon how much you want to spend. Just remember though, they all do the same job of bringing colored light into the body cells to promote healing.

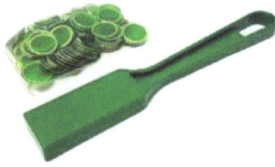

- A Magnetic wand can be used to balance the meridians and is easily obtained on Amazon. http://www.amazon.com/Green-Magnetic-Piece-Bingo-Markers/dp/B003JSTVRI/ref=sr_1_1?ie=UTF8&qid=1458598325&sr=8-1&keywords=bingo+wand+magnetic

So, as you can see there are choices available depending upon whether or not the price is right.

APPENDIX 3: DENTAL CONNECTION

When a particular tooth is troublesome and painful, look to the related meridian for an allergy or imbalance, since some of the major meridians pass through the gum and dental areas. From the chart, pinpointing the sensitive tooth reveals the meridian pair that is unbalanced. Use the appropriate color directly on the affected tooth, and balance the associated meridian using AcuColors technique in Section 3. Section III: Balancing the Meridians

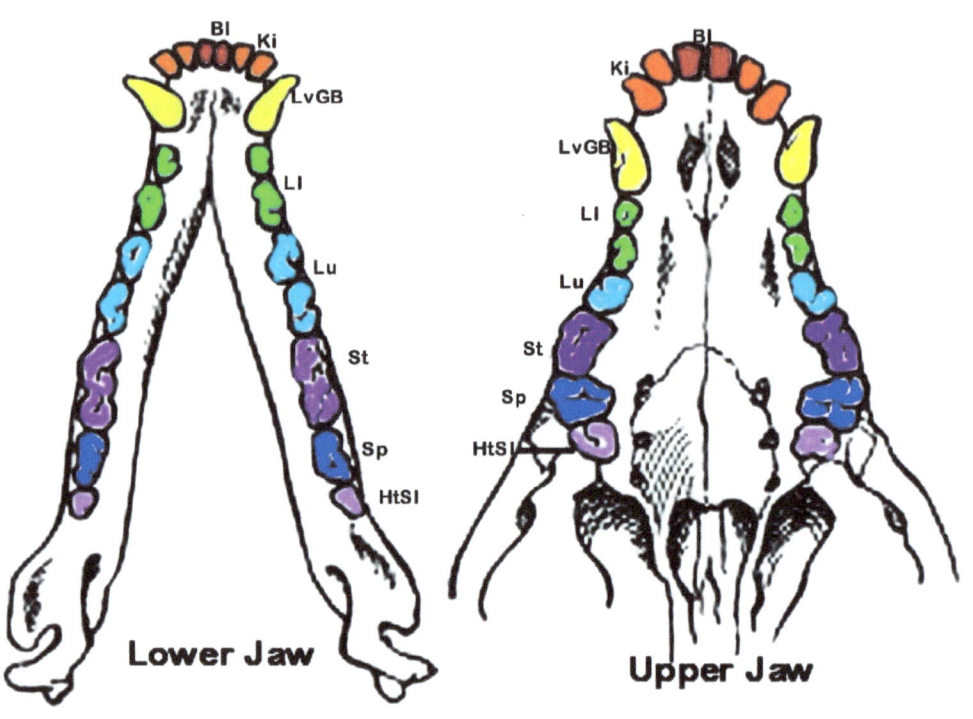

TEETH	MERIDIAN	COLOR
Front Incisors	Bladder	Red
Lateral Incisors	Kidney	Orange
Cuspids	Liver/GB	Yellow
Bicuspids	Large Intestine	Green
Premolars	Lung	Turquoise
Molars	Stomach	Violet
Molars	Spleen	Indigo Blue
Molars	Heart/S	UV

APPENDIX 2: EFFECTS OF COLOR

1. When applied to the acupoints of the body, Color penetrates deeper into the cells allowing more healing, than does acupuncture.
2. Increases blood capillary circulation and vascular activity by promoting improvement in the metabolism of nitric oxide (NO). This facilitates improved regulation of vasodilation and leads to the formation of new capillaries - this in turn provides additional oxygen and nutrients to accelerate natural tissue healing processes and eventually evokes a cascade of beneficial biochemical processes.
3. Stimulates synthesis of adenosine tri-phosphate (ATP)—an immediate energy source for muscle contraction and essential in the metabolism of all cellular processes and sustaining living systems
4. Relaxes muscles, reduces nerve excitability and stimulates nerve transmission
5. Reduces scar tissue and stimulates wound healing
6. Increases lymphatic system activity and relieves edema and discomfort associated with swelling
7. Stimulates acupuncture points and immune response
8. Stimulates production of collagen—the most important component of wound healing
9. Increases phagocytosis - the body's natural process to scavenge dead and degenerated cells and is important to the infection control process required for healing
10. Increases RNA/DNA synthesis - this stimulates cellular reproduction and facilitates accelerated replacement of damaged cells
11. Increases production of endorphins from the brain - promoting pain reduction and mood elevation
12. Stimulates production of adrenals— which facilitate long term pain relief and resilience to stress.
13. Reduces inflammation and swelling in chronic conditions of arthritis, bursitis, and tendonitis
14. Stimulates fibroblastic activity - promoting repair of connective tissue and formation of collagen fibers
15. Stimulates tissue granulation and connective tissue formation - an important process in the healing of wounds, ulcers and inflamed tissues.[iii]

The following chart outlines each color and its benefits to the body.

Red

Red reduces *inflammation and pain*. Brings warmth, energy and stimulation, therefore good for energy, fatigue, colds, chilly and passive people. Red energizes heart and blood circulation, it builds up the blood and heightens a low blood pressure. Energizes all organs and the senses hearing, smell, taste, vision and touch. Increases sexual desire and activity. Stimulates ovulation and menstruation. Never treat cancer with red, because this color will stimulate cell growth!

Red links with and stimulates the root chakra, at the base of the spine, causing the adrenal glands to release adrenalin. This results in greater strength. Red causes hemoglobin to multiply, thus increasing energy and raising body temperature. It is excellent for anemia and blood-related conditions. It loosens, opens up clogs, releases stiffness and constrictions. It is excellent for areas that have become stiffened or constricted. Do not use on Cancer cells!

Orange

Orange is warm, cheering, non-constricting and brings *joy*. Orange has a freeing action upon the body and mind, relieving repressions. Orange shows new possibilities and other options in life. Stimulates creative thinking and enthusiasm, and helps assimilate new ideas. It is also helpful in dealing with excess sexual expression.

Orange stimulates the lungs, the respiration and the digestion. Increases the activity of the thyroid. Relieves muscle cramps and spasms. Increases the amount of mother milk.

Finally, orange links very strongly with the sacral chakra.

Yellow

Yellow *moves a sluggish lymphatic system*. It helps strengthen the nerves and the mind. It helps awaken mental inspiration and stimulates higher mentality. Thus, it is an excellent color for nervous or nerve-related conditions or ailments. It also energizes the muscles. Dark yellow soothes pains in the nerves (shooting pains)

Yellow can be used for conditions of the stomach, liver, and intestines. Speeds up the digestion and assimilation, and the stool.

It helps the pores of the skin and aids scarred tissue in healing itself.

Yellow links with and stimulates the solar plexus, or psychic center. It can be used for psychic burnout or other psychic-related conditions or ailments. Activates and cheers up depressed and melancholic people. Gives lust for life.

Green

Green is the color of Nature and the earth. It is balance and harmony in essence and possesses a soothing influence upon both mind and body. It is neither relaxing nor astringent in its impact. Green can be used for just about any condition in need of healing.

Green rings psychological and emotional harmony and balance.

Green links with and stimulates the heart chakra. Green affects blood pressure and all conditions of the heart. It has both an energizing effect and a moderating or soothing effect.

It cures hormonal imbalances. Stimulates growth hormone and rejuvenation. Cleans and purifies from germs, bacteria and rotting material. Harmonizes the digestion, stomach, liver, gall. Has a healing effect on kidneys. Increases immunity. Builds up muscles, bones and tissues. Stimulates inner peace. Strengthens nervous system. Green is most often used for *infections*.

Turquoise

Turquoise cools down inflammations (don't forget rheumatic inflammations), fever, high blood pressure, stops bleedings, reliefs the bursting headaches, calms strong emotions like anger, aggression or hysteria. Brings tranquility. Anti-itching. Anti-irritation (for instance redness of the skin), anti-stress. Soothes suffering.

Turquoise can be used for any type of ailments associated with speech, communication, or the throat. Excellent for laryngitis or inflammation of the larynx.

Turquoise *links with the subconscious* and stimulates the throat chakra. The throat chakra is often referenced as the "power center" and "the greatest center in the body" because it is the primary center of expression and communication, through speech.

Blue

Blue is *sedating*, calming, cooling, electric, astringent. Dr. Edwin Babbitt, in his classic, "The Principles of Light and Color," states that "The Blue Ray is one of the greatest antiseptics in the world."

Blue is a great purifier of the bloodstream and also benefits mental problems. It is a freeing and purifying agent.

Blue combines the deep blue of devotion with a trace of stabilizing and objective red. Blue is cool, electric, and astringent.

Blue links with and stimulates the brow chakra (third eye) and controls the pineal gland. It governs both physical and spiritual perception. It can be of great assistance in dealing with ailments of the eyes and ears.

Violet

These are colors of transformation. They heal melancholy, hysteria, delusions and alcohol addiction and bring spiritual insights and renewal.

These colors slow down an over-active heart; stimulate the spleen and the white blood cells (immunity). Bring *sleep*. Soothe mental and emotional stress. Decrease sexual activity. Decrease sensitivity to pain. They help in detoxification.

Leonardo da Vinci proclaimed that you can increase the power of meditation ten-fold by meditating under the gentle rays of Violet, as found in Church windows.

APPENDIX 6: PET CPR & FIRST AID

Recognizing & Responding to an Emergency

- ❏ Check the scene around the animal, collect info—poisoning? objects?
- ❏ Cautiously approach, restrain & capture an injured animal—blanket or towel
- ❏ Check the animal for responsiveness and pulse at inner thigh over black dot.
- ❏ Treating emergencies— Breathing, Trauma, Bleeding.

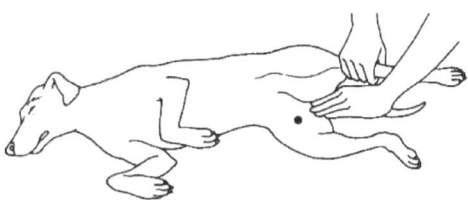

Starting CPR and Rescue Breathing

A = AIRWAY: Open the airway and remove any visible objects from the mouth.

- **Choking-most common reason dogs stop breathing**– food, toys or trauma, tongue swelling from allergy; poison
- **Signs of choking**—raspy loud noise or cough upon exhale; gag or retch; rapid shallow breathing, outward stretching of head; **pale or blue gums**; physical distress, panic, collapse, LOC
- **Conscious Choking**:
    1. Finger sweep debris from mouth.

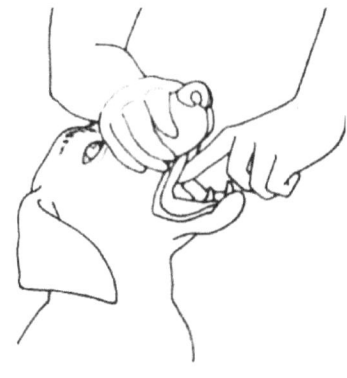

87

2. Grab pet by back legs with head down if pet is still coughing, till object out.

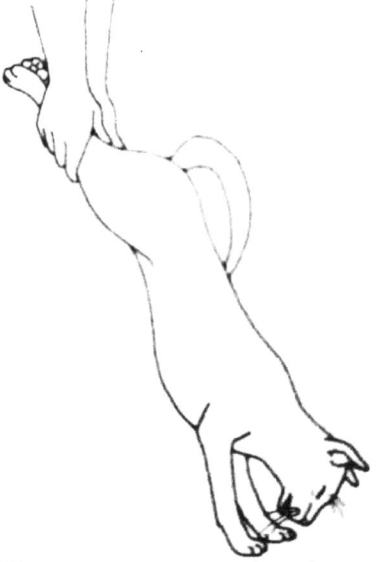

3. Place arms around waist, make a fist and do abdominal thrusts 5x.

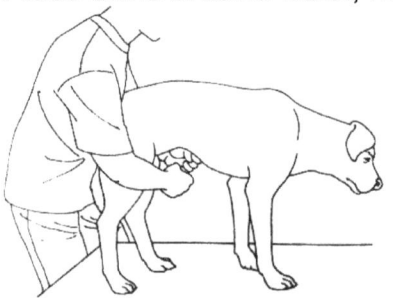

4. Add back blows if necessary.

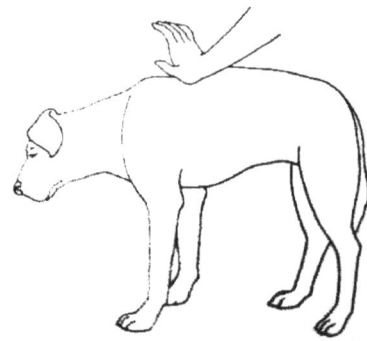

5. Check airway by extending head & neck & pull tongue forward. Repeat steps 1-4 until airway is clear, then continue with rescue breaths.

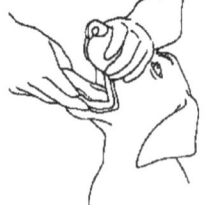

B = **BREATHING**:

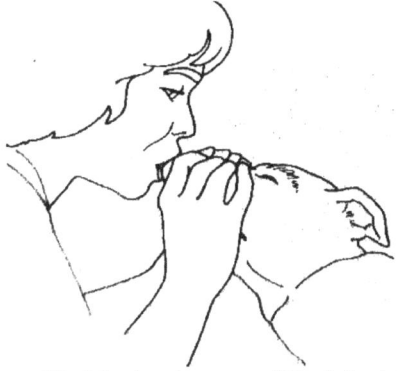

- Pet is laying on **Right** side. **Left** heart side up.
- Look Listen Feel for breathing for 10 sec
- Once airway cleared, close mouth & lips w/one hand
- Place mouth over pet's nose & breathe 1 sec. after 4-5 breaths, check for breath, if none, continue at rate of 15-20 bpm

C = CIRCULATION

- Find femoral pulse or heart rate, if none…

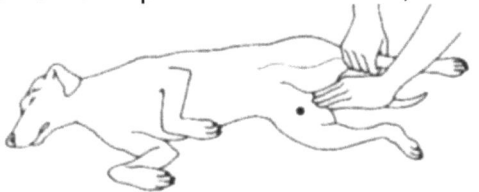

- Do 15 compressions to 2 breaths

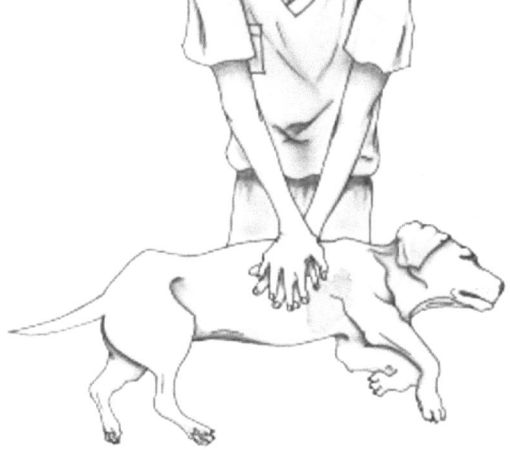

- Use 2 Hands for Large; 1 Hand for Small

APPENDIX 4: SPINAL CONNECTION

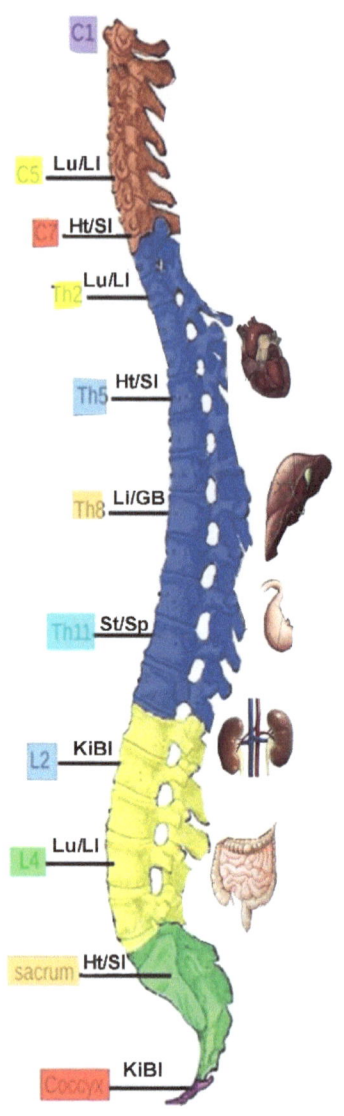

SPINE Location	EMOTIONS
C1-C4	Occipital HA- Meningitis Fear, anxiety & aggression, confusion
C5-C6 Lu/LI	Zone of Melancholy Afraid of humiliation Lacks flexibility
C7-T1 Ht/SI	Fearful/closed heart, easily hurt.
T2-T4 Lu/LI	Emotional scars from old wounds.
T5-T7 Ht/SI	Converter pt for T4&T5
T8-T10 Lv/GB	Vertebrae of transformation. Easily angry & irritable
T11-L1 St/Sp	One of psych zones. Worry
L2-L3 Ki/Bl	Subconscious pain and fear
L4-L5 Lu/LI	L5 Connects to thyroid. Aggressive male.
Sacrum Ht/SI	Oppressed. Loss of power. Suppressed emotion.
Coccyx	Zone of emotions, fear & phobias.

APPENDIX 5: GROOMING GUIDE

Seriously consider grooming your own pet. It's not as difficult as many people think, but it does take time—probably about an hour each month, plus 20-30 minutes each week. Grooming is beneficial because it allows special bonding and assessment time, and it is very cost effective. One month of grooming cost (about $60-80) will pay for a new set of clippers.

Most short-haired animals need very little grooming because their hair doesn't mat as easily as the long-haired ones. I've learned from experience that although no shedding of fur, those special poodle-mix breeds, unfortunately do need to be groomed on a regular basis, since their hair mats easily around the ears, hindquarters, and underarms. But, no problem… if I can learn to groom on my own, then so can you!

Start Grooming your pet while he is still young; that way he will think that it is just part of his normal routine. In spite of any resistance, he does like the attention you given him, so don't give up. I made plenty of "whoops" boo-boos, but thank goodness, it grows out! Here's a great website: http://pets.wahl.com/grooming-tips/

The Grooming Routine
- BRUSHING: long-haired pets daily to prevent mats. Brush fur before clipping or bathing pet. This is also a good time to assess the condition of the body. Are there hotspots, matted fur, patches of hair loss, fleas, ticks, ear mites, cracked or broken nails?

- CLIPPING: Obtain a good set of hair clippers—Andis, Oster, Wahl. When well maintained through proper cleaning and oiling they should last for 10-20 years. Most sets include various guards to the length of fur desired. For cold winter months use #2 (6mm) or #3 (10mm); for summer months use #1 (3mm). When trimming hold the clipper guard perpendicular to the fur and move slowly down the body from head to tail. Going against the nap of the fur will cut shorter. You may want to take off the guard around the feet and legs. When your pet goes outside and walks in the mud, he tracks it inside if the fur is not trimmed around the top and bottom of the paws.

- TRIMMING: Prevent hair mats by trimming hair short behind ears, on underside around legs, anus, and urethra. Clip fur once a week around eyes, ears and feet so that it's not such a big job once a month. Check ears for mites, and other pests. Keep hairs trimmed around ears to prevent intruders from invading.

- BATHING: Bathing or Showering pet inside during winter is much preferred. Adjust water temperature and work shampoo into lather from head to toe. If your pet has a tendency to scratch and chew on his hindquarters, use an oatmeal shampoo, even with lidocaine for stubborn itching and sores. Add Omega 3 & 6 powder to food, or give as a chew. This has done wonders for my own dog who used to visit the Vet monthly for cortisone shots since he would chew himself raw over one little flea or bite.

- NAILS: Obtain a safe and painless nail trimmer. I have an Oster pair ($5). Trim nails & dewclaws about once a month. Trim only the clear portion staying away from the white opaque quick which will bleed. If accidentally cut, apply a styptic powder to stop bleeding. Dewclaws if not trimmed, will grow and embed into the skin.
- TEETH: Brush teeth daily or at least once a week. Keep teeth free of tartar buildup by giving them a daily milkbone or a rawhide bone. Use baking soda never fluoridated toothpaste on a toothbrush.

Just think of your pet as one of your kids and you will see the necessity of doing your own grooming out of love and concern for your pet's health and well-being.

GLOSSARY

ABBREVIATION	TRANSLATION	EXPLANATION
Acupoints	Acupuncture Points	These are specific meridian points used to repair damage.to the body.
AI	Autoimmune disease	Cells attack & destroy their own body cells Ex: MG, SLE, RA.
ANS	Autonomic Nervous System	Automatic body functions controlled by the Medulla Oblongata.
BL	Bladder	Meridian from each eye down the Spine to the outside of each back paw.
CV	Conception Vessel	Central Meridian up Front of the Body.
DDD	Degen Disc Disease	Degenerative Disc Disease of the Spine
ECIWO	Every cell in Everything	Embryo Containing Info of Whole Organism.
EFT	Emotional Freedom Technique	Releases emotions by tapping on meridian points.
FW	Finger Width	Uses a person's finger width to measure the distance from various sites to find acupoints on his/her body.
GB	Gall Bladder	Meridian from each eye around each ear and down each side to the 4th toe.
GI	Gastrointestinal	Pertaining to Stomach & Abdomen.
GV	Governing Vessel	Central Meridian up the Spine over the head to the upper lip.
HA	Headache	Migraine, Sinus, or other Headaches.
↑HR	Heart rate	Faster heart rate or pulse
Ht	Heart	Meridian from each armpit down to 5th finger.
Ki	Kidney	Meridian from middle of back paw up the Body
LBP	Low Back Pain	Pain in the Lumbar-Sacral region of the Back.
L	Left	Left side of body
L2	Lumbar disc 2	Lumbar vertebrae location on the spine
L5	Lumbar disc 5	
LH	Left Hand	Finger 1=Thumb; 2=Index; 3=Middle; 4=Ring; 5=Little.
LI	Large Intestine	Meridian from each thumb up the arm to the nose.
LOC	Unconscious	Loss of Consciousness
Lu	Lung	Meridian down each arm of the Body.
Lv	Liver	Meridian from each big toe up to the chest of the Body.
MG	Myasthenia Gravis	Weakness of the Muscles. May start in the eyelids or eyes & progress to lungs
MS	Multiple Sclerosis	Auto Immune system destroys myelin sheath covering nerves.

NLR	Neurolymphatic Reflex Points	When stimulated with a warm color these reflex points energize, remove toxins, clear negative energy from the meridian system, and balance the meridians and their related organs. Or, when treated with a cool color they can sedate.
N-M	Nerve-Muscle	The N-M system is where most of degeneration occurs.
NV pt	NeuroVascular holding point	These points are used in acupressure for various health issues.
N/V	Nausea/Vomiting	Gastrointestinal symptoms.
NP	Neck Pain	Pain in the upper torso, Shoulder & Neck region of the Body.
PC	Pericardium	Meridian up the middle of each Arm. Pericardium is the tissue around the heart; so this meridian governs heart function and also reproductive function.
RA	Rheumatoid Arthritis	Autoimmune disease where the joints are attacked.
R	Right	Right side of body
RH	Right Hand	Finger 1=Thumb; 2=Index; 3=Middle; 4=Ring; 5=Little.
↑RR	Respiratory rate	
SI	Small Intestine	Meridian from the 5th fingers up the arm to each ear.
SLE	Systemic Lupus Erythematosus	Auto Immune system attacks the body tissues. Butterfly rash is characteristic.
SOB	Shortness of Breath	Difficulty breathing.
Sp	Spleen	Meridian from the Ball of the back paw up the Body.
St	Stomach	Meridian from the nose down each side of the Body to big toes.
Sx	Sign or Symptom	Description of what you observe in your pet.
TB	Tuberculosis	Scrofula is a condition of TB that affects the lymph nodes.
TCM	Traditional Chinese Medicine	Eastern Medicine that treats the whole person in Body-Soul-Spirit.
TW	Triple Warmer	Meridian up the middle of each Arm. Governs glandular function.
♪	Notes	Alternative ideas that complement therapy.
💧	Drop of oil	Tips on use of Essential Oils
🦶	Footnote	Foot Reflexology Tips for Back Paws

REFERENCES

Healing Touch for Dogs e-book by Dr. Michael W. Fox, Newmarket Press, NY.

Acu-Cat: A Guide to Feline Acupressure e-book by Amy Snow & Nancy Zidonis, 2nd ed., Tallgrass Pub, CO. 2012

Color Therapy for Animals e-book by Julianne Bien, Spectrahue Light & Sound Inc., Canada. 2014.

The Canine Acupressure Workbook e-book by Lisa B. Speaker & JoMarie Indovina, Dogma Inc, CO. 2012.

Energy Medicine e-book by Donna Eden & David Feinstein, the Penguin Group, NY. 2008.

Essential Oils for Your Pet e-book by Kathleen Kalaf, 2015.

The Healing Code by Alexander Loyd, PhD, ND, Publisher: Grand Central Life & Style. 2011, pg. 157.

Emotion Code, by Dr. Bradley Nelson, ebook, Well Unmasked Publishing, 2007.

www.chinalifeweb.com *Which Tongue Are You?*

Grooming tips *http://pets.wahl.com/grooming-tips/*

The Blissful Dog *https://theblissfuldog.com/aligning-dogs-chakras/*

---

[i] http://www.soundessence.net/meridians.php   The Meridian Connection

www.ingramcontent.com/pod-product-compliance
Lightning Source LLC
Chambersburg PA
CBHW051021180526
45172CB00002B/427